Brain Death

Science and Society:
A Purdue University Series in Science,
Technology, and Human Values

Leon E. Trachtman, General Editor

Volume 5

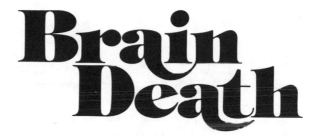

Brain Death

Ethical Considerations

by Douglas N. Walton

Purdue University
West Lafayette, Indiana
1980

Any opinions, findings, conclusions, or recommendations expressed herein are those of the author
and do not necessarily reflect the views of the Social Science and Humanities Research Council of
Canada or of the University of Winnipeg.

Second printing, April 1981

Library of Congress Card Catalog Number 80-80845
International Standard Book Number 0-931682-12-6
Printed in the United States of America

For Karen

Contents

Acknowledgments

I would like to acknowledge support by research
grants from the Social Sciences and Humanities Research Council of Canada and the University of Winnipeg. Dr. Michael Newman has been particularly
helpful, giving the insights of a practising neurologist in discussions and in helpful comments on an
earlier draft of this manuscript. Dr. Robert Veatch
also reviewed that previous draft and made numerous
corrections, comments, and suggestions that have
been gratefully taken into account. Numerous discussions with Mr. Harvey Fleming have contributed
at many points.

The active cooperation of the Health Sciences
Center Library, the Law Library of the University
of Manitoba, and the Interloan Service of the University of Winnipeg has been greatly appreciated.
I am very grateful to Mrs. Amy Merrett for her
punctilious typing and proofreading.

Part One

Criteria for Determining Brain Death

Introduction

This monograph is a survey and evaluation of the arguments for and against equating the death of a person with the irreversible destruction of brain function (brain death). The traditional understanding has been to equate the death of the person with irreversible cessation of cardiorespiratory function, indicated, for example by the absence of pulse, breathing, or heartbeat. Our conclusion will be that the new equation is defensible in that cogent arguments for it exist and that no existing refutation is conclusive or cannot be met with rebuttals, provided we mean by *brain death* irreversible destruction of the whole brain including the subcortex. We will also raise a number of pointed, open questions that the brain death exponent[1] needs to answer, thereby suggesting that the attempted refutations raise some significant unresolved issues of concern.

The primary arguments tend to fall into three main classes: the so-called practical issues of need for organ transplantation, need for reduction of socioeconomic burdens, need for protection of transplant surgeons and other health care personnel; philosophical arguments that brain death corresponds, or does not, to what is essential to the concept of the death of a person; ethical arguments that the loss of personhood consequent on a declaration of brain death can either lead to ethical

1

abuse or that not so declaring would be a moral
error.

The form of one worrisome kind of argument
against brain death has the form of the slippery
slope: If we allow a declaration of brain death,
it is argued, this will lead to keeping ventilated,
warm, and pulsing brain-dead cadavers around as
storage units for organs or chemicals or even for
experiments. We will evaluate this argument very
carefully and show why it does, indeed, need to be
handled with care and why it has features that can
be seriously misleading. Although this argument
does raise highly significant issues about the
treatment of cadavers, I will argue that it does
not decisively overturn the equation of death with
brain death, provided the brain death exponent can
satisfactorily explain why human bodies should
be treated with respect, particularly newly dead
bodies with continuing cardiorespiratory function.

Another form of argument we examine is the charge
that the medical diagnostic criteria for brain death
are not certain enough to safely rule out the possibility of life. Here we argue that if we take
brain death to comprise only the destruction of the
cerebral hemispheres or any other single part of
the brain, then the notion is open to reservations
on grounds of safety, but that there do exist sets
of criteria for whole-brain death that are not open
to any well-documented counterexamples or overwhelm-
ing counterarguments that have been advanced at the
present time to the author's knowledge, and that
seem to have reasonable presumption of safety. Thus,
we prefer whole-brain death to a notion of brain
death based on the irreversible destruction of any
part of the brain, even the cerebrum.

As well as looking at medical-diagnostic criteria,
we examine the more purely philosophical arguments
for and against the equation of death and brain
death. We look at the cardiorespiratory concept to
determine whether it is the circulation of fluids

that is central or the spontaneity of circulation.
And we will encounter some conceptual arguments that
the brain-oriented conception has primacy over the
cardiorespiratory conception.

Next we look at the philosophical arguments that
attempt to establish the brain death equation by
finding some essential indicator of life or personhood, e.g. mental activity, such that (a) the irreversible cessation of this indicator may be called
death, and (b) this indicator coincides with brain
function. In this area we will find that some
worthwhile proposals have been made, but in the
absence of their clearer articulation and in the
absence of necessary work on the philosophical
analysis of the concept of death, these arguments
have reasonable presumption but are hardly thought
of as conclusive at present.

Another question is the precise physical location and extent of the area of the brain and its
environs to be considered in brain death, a concern
that predominates in part three.

The significance of brain death as a concept is
occasioned by the well-known life-prolonging dilemmas brought about by the fact that it is possible
to continue cardiorespiratory functions by mechani-
cal means, even while the brain has deteriorated to
a point clearly incompatible with the possibility
of any return of conscious awareness. The proposed
advantages of a declaration of death in such a situation are that effort, emotional exhaustion, finan-
cial burdens, and an unsettling situation for all
involved can be alleviated by sparing a futile pro-
longation of treatment. Second, a declaration of
brain death could, in many cases, facilitate favourable possibilities of organ transplantation. Third,
legislation making such a declaration of death
possible could remove many ethical and legal uncertainties. But what are the potential disadvan-
tages? If death is equated with brain death, it
would follow in the opinion of many that a ventilated brain-dead cadaver is just that, a *corpse*

without rights, perhaps an object for unthinking
experimentation or callous treatment. Moreover,
any remote possibility that anyone declared brain
dead could still be consciously aware or potentially returnable to life is a worrisome factor that
calls for great caution in understanding and determining brain death.

These are the most basic and widely cited arguments for or against. But, as we will see, there
are others. And these basic arguments have numerous variations and subarguments.

Legal Developments

How are we to deal ethically with cases in which
cardiorespiratory function is provided artifically
by machines and in which we seem, reasonably, to
want to sanction removal of the machine? There are
two different philosophical avenues of ethical approach to the life-prolonging dilemmas and in many
situations they converge. One approach is to say
of some machine-sustained individuals that they are
dead (i.e., brain dead) if their state is incompatible with brain function, even if the traditional
cardiorespiratory functions are present. The other
approach is to say that even though such a person
may be, in some sense, alive, they or their next
of kin or guardian may be allowed to exercise the
right to refuse treatment. Consequently, the medical staff may reduce or withdraw aggressive therapy,
for example, by removing the ventilator. The two
kinds of cases are conceptually distinct, but it is
worth noting that they sometimes overlap in reality
and that some would argue for removing a ventilator
on grounds of the permissibility of withdrawing
therapy while disagreeing that this may be done because death (brain death) has occurred, while others
might argue for the same action on grounds of brain
death.

Bringing in the concept of whole-brain death will
not solve the vast majority of cases in which the
question has arisen of whether or not withdrawal of
therapy or "allowing to die" is permissible. In a
majority of these kinds of cases--as some of my own
initial studies in a pilot project at the intensive
care ward at Saint Boniface Hospital have indi-
cated--brain death is not at issue. The discussion
between Veatch and others (Annals of the New York
Academy of Sciences, vol. 315, 1978, p. 337) also
supports this observation. At any rate, the concept of brain death would not apply to these other
cases unless it were stretched to a point where
almost nobody in the serious literature I am familiar with would be presently prepared to stretch it.
We will see, however, that making the move from
whole-brain death to cerebral death (destruction
of the cerebral hemispheres only) would expand the
number of ethically significant cases covered by
brain death legislation.

Ways of dealing with these ethical decisions vary
from hospital to hospital, but these two approaches
are usually distinguished. For example, Dr. Michael Newman of Saint Boniface Hospital finds that
as a neurologist he is asked to determine death
in two circumstances. The first is the case in
which the patient is felt to be in a moribund state
and the attending physician either does not want
to use the respirator or would like to take the
patient off the respirator. He reports (personal
communication, 1979) that he does not try to solve
this problem by defining death at all, but by trying to determine whether the respirator is a useful means of treatment. The question is one of the
discontinuation of therapy, whether the respirator
is going to cure disease or whether, in all reasonable probability, the underlying disease is going
to result in death without return to consciousness.
That is the decision to be made by the patient--if
he is conscious--his next of kin, and the physicians. The second circumstance occurs when the

patient is wanted as an organ donor, and it is
here that the concept of brain death can be useful.

Not every physician might divide the two sets
of circumstances in precisely the same way as Dr.
Newman has, but the underlying separation of the
brain death issue and the discontinuation of therapy issue in the decision-making framework is virtually universal in hospital practice. Particulars
may vary, but the two basic avenues of ethical approach are distinct.

These two approaches are evident in trends toward recent legislation in Canada, as in other
countries. The Natural Death Act, presently being
discussed by a committee of the Ontario legislature,
proposes that a person be allowed to make the following direction to his attending physician and
medical staff:

> I, . . ., being of sound mind, willfully and volun-
> tarily, direct that all life-sustaining procedures
> be withheld or withdrawn if at any time I should
> be in a terminal condition and where the applica-
> tion of life-sustaining procedures would serve
> only to artificially prolong the moment of death.

What is a "terminal condition" is left to physicians to determine. The philosophical basis of
this proposal is not that a person in a terminal
condition is already dead, i.e., no longer a person. Rather, the idea is that such a person, by
indicating a wish to exercise his right to refuse
treatment, can santion the withdrawal of therapy
that will result in death.[2]

At the federal level, the approach of withdrawal
of therapy is being considered, and, as we will see,
the Law Reform Commission has made recommendations
on brain death legislation. Yet, at the provincial
level, the brain death approach has already been
enacted upon.

The Province of Manitoba has adopted a statutory
definition of death which equates the death of a

person with brain death (Manitoba Law Reform Commission, 1974). The definition if formulated as
follows:

> For all purposes within the legislative competence
> of the Legislature of Manitoba the death of a per-
> son takes place at the time at which irreversible
> cessation of all that person's brain function oc-
> curs.

It would appear from the Report of the Law Reform
Commission that this remarkably advanced piece of
legislation was, to a great extent, inspired by the
work of Dr. Michael G. Saunders. The report is
very cautious in a number of ways, stressing the
inviolability of the human person and the care
needed "lest undue or erroneous reliance be placed
on machine techniques which are fundamentally lab-
oratory procedures" (p. 20). Care in diagnosing
drug overdose cases, for example, is stressed. The
report does not direct itself to the question of
feasibility of diagnosis, however. Rather, the aim
is to produce a fair and accurate definition of
death that will preserve human rights (p. 21).

Similarly, in the United States, acts granting
individuals permission to direct their physicians
to reduce or withdraw therapy in case of terminal
illness have been passed.[3] At the same time, many
states have adopted brain death legislation, as we
will see.

Here our exclusive concern will be with brain
death, but the reader should be aware of this other
possible legislative avenue that could be of assis-
tance in some of the same problems.

There has been considerable disagreement over
whether a brain-oriented definition of death should
be legislated as a statutory provision. Objections
are that a statute might be too inflexible or would
require too many amendments and that it presupposes
medical and philosophical unanimity which does not
exist. Skegg (1976) counters that legislation could

have advantages. It is doubtful, he suggests
(p. 191), that the matter is best dealt with in the
course of a particular dispute. The particular
circumstances of the case at issue may be given dis-
proportionate weight, and litigants would have to
go through tiresome and expensive court proceedings to get a decision.

To be sure, genuinely constructive and clear
legislation would have decisive advantages, but it
presupposes that determinations based on the legislation can be made precisely and without unethical
consequences. But there seems to be widespread
public confusion and doubt about the concept of
brain death. Are the medical criteria safe, so
there can be no possibility of a living person declared dead? And do we understand the concept of
death clearly enough at the philosophical level to
build a definition of it into legislation? The
questions are still very much open for ethical discussion, but brain death legislation is moving
rapidly into effect.

Two kinds of cases, in particular, indicate the
necessity for a legal definition of death. First,
there are disputed cases of inheritance. In the
case of *Thomas v Anderson* (1950; 215 p 2d 478), the
question was whether two joint tenants died simul-
taneously. If so, their property would be divided
equally. If not, it would pass to the heir of the
"survivor." The other kind of case is that in
which a doctor who ceases treatment in order to
transplant a brain-dead donor's organ might be
charged with homicide. An example is the Virginia
case of *Tucker v Lower*, in which the defendant's
brother charged that the physician who turned the
respirator off and transplanted the brain-dead patient's heart was guilty of unlawful homicide. The
jury ruled in favour of the defendant medical team,
however.[4]

In a 1975 Massachusetts case, the defendant's
lawyer, relying on the traditional definition of
death (cessation of circulation, respiration, and

all bodily functions), claimed that the action of
the physicians and the family in taking a brain-
dead murder victim off the respirator deprived the
defendant of a defense, for, if the victim had lived
a year and a day after his assault, even though on
a respirator, the defendant could not be charged
with homicide.[5]

At any rate, we can see why there is some legal
impetus to redefine death in terms of loss of brain
function and replace the traditional cardiorespiratory notion of the law.

In the Quinlan case, there was not an adequate
medical basis for raising the issue of brain death.
Rather, the question was one of whether withdrawal
of the "extraordinary care" procedures could be removed by permission of the legal guardian. Dr. Julius Korein, who performed an examination of Karen
Quinlan, makes clear in a comment (*Annals of the
New York Academy of Sciences*, vol. 315, p. 320f.,
"Editor's Comment"), that she was not brain-dead,
nor was she ever pronounced brain-dead. She was in
a "persistent vegetative state" with no evidence of
cognitive function, but did exhibit a "complex rep-
ertoire of reflexes", electroencephalograph (EEG)
activity, and normal intracranial blood circulation.[6]

The brain death legislation falls into three
different types of statements. The first kind is
exemplified by the Kansas statute enacted in 1970.

> (1) A person will be considered medically and legal-
> ly dead if, in the opinion of a physician,
> based on ordinary standards of medical practice,
> there is the absence of spontaneous respiratory
> and cardiac function and, because of the dis-
> ease or condition which caused, directly or
> indirectly, these functions to cease, or be-
> cause of the passage of time since these func-
> tions ceased, attempts at resuscitation are
> considered hopeless; and, in this event, death
> will have occurred at the time these functions
> ceased; or

(2) A person will be considered medically and legally dead if, in the opinion of a physician,
based on ordinary standards of medical practice, there is the absence of spontaneous brain
function; and if based on ordinary standards
of medical practice, during reasonable attempts
to either maintain or restore spontaneous circulatory or respiratory function in the absence
of aforesaid brain function, it appears that
further attempts at resuscitation or supportive
maintenance will not succeed, death will have
occured at the time when these conditions first
coincide. Death is to be pronounced before
artificial means of supporting respiratory and
circulatory function are terminated and before
any vital organ is removed for purposes of
transplantation.

Maryland passed an identical statute in 1972 and a
similar law was passed in Virginia in 1973. Other
states adopting this type of proposal are New
Mexico (1973), Alaska (1974), and Oregon (1975).
The Kansas model has often been criticized because
it appears to postulate two different definitions
of death--a pluralism that many have found to be
an intuitively unfortunate sin against public psychology (as the Law Reform Commission of Canada,
1979, p. 43, put it). The problem is that it appears to suggest that a transplant donor could be
considered "dead" earlier than a nondonor, even if
both were in exactly the same condition.
    In the sequel, however, I will suggest that the
Kansas statute need not be interpreted this way at
all, despite its own mention of "alternative definitions of death." It could be interpreted as
leaving the question of the concept of death open,
while formulating two sets of criteria for death.
So interpreted, the pluralism of the Kansas formu-
lation need not seem quite so potentially alarm-
ing.
    The second kind of statement is the Capron and
Kass (1972) proposal.

> A person will be considered dead if in the an-
> nounced opinion of a physician, based on ordinary
> standards of medical practice, he has experienced
> an irreversible cessation of spontaneous respira-
> tory and circulatory functions. In the event that
> artificial means of support preclude a determina-
> tion that these functions have ceased, a person
> will be considered dead if in the announced opin-
> ion of a physician, based on ordinary standards of
> medical practice, he has experienced an irrevers-
> ible cessation of spontaneous brain functions.
> Death will have occurred at the time when the rele-
> vant functions ceased.

This proposal makes it quite clear that two criteria
for determination of death are being postulated and,
thus, avoids the suspicion of conceptual pluralism.
In addition, it removes further uncertainties of
application by specifying the circumstances under
which the brain-related criteria are to be used.
States that have adopted legislation based on the
Capron-Kass statement are Michigan (1975), West
Virginia (1975), Louisiana (1976), Iowa (1976), and
Montana (1977).

The third type of statement, that of the American Bar Association (ABA), adopted by its House of
Delegates in 1975, is simple and direct: "For all
legal purposes, a human body with irreversible
cessation of total brain function, according to
usual and customary standards of medical practice,
shall be considered dead." A criticism of this
type of proposal is that it entirely fails to mention the cardiorespiratory criteria still widely
in use. The response of its defenders--see Veith
el al. (1977, p. 1748) is that the practice is to
only declare death if breathing and heartbeat have
ceased long enough to assure brain death. Thus,
it is said that the statute at least implicitly
recognizes the traditional criteria.

The ABA statute is the basis of legislation in
California (1974), Georgia (1975), Idaho (1977),
and Tennessee (1976). With modifications, similar

statements form the core of statutes in Oklahoma
(1975), Illinois (1975), and Oregon (1975).

In 1977 the Law Reform Commission of Australia
issued a Report on Transplantation proposing a definition that stated that a person could be considered
dead in the case of total and irreversible cessation of all vital brain functions. The report also
states that death could be determined on the basis
of the arrest of spontaneous respiratory and cardiac
functions. Initially, this statement seems similar
to the ABA proposal, but the addition of cardiorespiratory criteria for certain circumstances makes
it much closer to the Capron-Kass model.

Similarly, the proposal put forward by the Law
Reform Commission of Canada (1979) is most like the
Capron-Kass model, because it adds clauses that
bring in cardiorespiratory criteria specifying the
circumstances in which each type of criterion is to
be applied.

> A person is dead when an irreversible cessation of
> all that person's brain functions has occurred.
>
> The cessation of brain functions can be determined
> by the prolonged absence of spontaneous cardiac
> and respiratory functions.
>
> When the determination of the absence of cardiac
> and respiratory functions is made impossible by
> the use of artificial means of support, the cessa-
> tion of the brain functions may be determined by
> any means recognized by the ordinary standards of
> current medical practice.

It is worthwhile to note that accompanying these
movements toward brain death legislation is a trend
toward legislation that would make it easier to remove organs for transplantation from a brain-dead
donor. At present--in the United States, for ex-
ample--surgeons must have a signed donor card or
obtain permission from the next of kin before organs
may be removed for transplantation.

On the other hand, removal of useful cadaver organs, e.g., pituitary glands for growth-hormone therapy, is routine hospital practice. Now a proposal has been put forward by Professor Jesse Dukeminier of the UCLA School of Law to make organ salvage routine unless there was a specific objection made by the person during his lifetime or unless the next of kin objects at the time of death.

According to Stuart (1977), the European Committee on Legal Cooperation in 1976 advocated two positions.

(1) It should be possible for removal of cadaver organs to be effected from the moment when it was established that the donor had irreversibly lost all his cerebral functions even though the functions of other organs might have been preserved.
(2) Legislation should move toward the adoption of presumed consent for removal of cadaver organs if circumstances give reason to believe that the family or the donor do not or would not have objected.

Thus, one can see how brain death legislation can be coupled with changing the legal status of burden of proof for permission of removal of cadaver organs for transplantation to change the legal circumstances of organ removal from brain-dead neomorts.

Medical Developments

Brain death is a term in emerging medical, legal, and common use that, as we will use it here, means complete destruction of the brain, irreversible cessation of the brain function.[7] The term is also a technical component of the medical vocabulary that is constantly evolving as more precise and sophisticated diagnostic criteria for determining brain death are being developed.

Walker (1974, p. 190) describes brain death medically as anoxic death of the high metabolizing

cerebral neurons. Five basic disturbances are at-
tendant: (1) failure of the blood-brain barrier,
(2) breakdown of neuronal membranes, (3) utilization
of oxygen below the level required for basic metab-
olism of nerve cells, (4) production and utilization of abnormal metabolic substances by the cells
(cannibalism), and (5) decrease or arrest of cerebral blood flow. As a result of the production of
these abnormal substances, the brain swells, even
further cutting off blood and oxygen, which, in
turn, leads to more rapid deterioration. For
further clinical descriptions see Black (1978),
Harp (1974), and Walker (1974).

In any inquiry of the sort here undertaken, some
will feel the issues are purely medical and others
purely philosophical. These presumptions are obstructive. Veatch (1975, p. 14) states that the
concept of death is "totally philosophical and in
no way a technical-medical issue." But Van Till
(1975, p. 137) says "[t]he diagnosis of death is
not in the last place a problem of definition." A
contradiction? No, because we must distinguish
between the concept of death and the diagnosis of
death. The analysis of the concept of death provides a target, an account of what it is that diagnostic criteria are thought to measure or determine.
Medical criteria for diagnosis are techniques for
determining, perhaps with some latitude of judgement required, when a specific patient may be said
to fall in the range marked off by the criteria.
The task is to attempt to correlate the philosophical and medical concepts and criteria.

Basic to understanding the controversy about
brain death is the development of new criteria for
its determination utilizing the electroencephalograph (EEG), a machine that registers electrical
activity in the brain. The "Report of the Ad Hoc
Committee of the Harvard Medical School to Examine
Brain Death" (Beecher, 1968) cites six criteria,
hereafter called the Harvard criteria: (1) unrecep-
tivity and unresponsiveness to external stimuli,

(2) no spontaneous muscular movement or spontaneous
breathing, (3) no reflexes, including brain and
spinal reflexes, (4) flat EEG, (5) all of the above
reverified after twenty-four hours, (6) patient not
to be hypothermic or under central nervous system
(CNS) depressants. A set of criteria subsequently
formulated by the University of Minnesota Health
Sciences Center (1971) is similar but places more
emphasis on clinical judgement and does not require
an EEG reading in all cases.[8]

The flat (isoelectric) EEG reading implies an
absence of biological activity of the brain cells,
since all living cells produce electrical activity.
There has been much discussion of the value and use
of the EEG in determining death.[9] Harp (1974,
p. 393) notes that according to a 1970 report of
the American Electroencephalographic Society, only
three of a study of 2,642 patients survived who
had a flat EEG reading. These three were drug overdose cases and would therefore fail to meet number 6
of the Harvard criteria.

Angiography is a technique that uses X-rays to
determine whether there is blood circulation in the
brain. A dye is injected into the carotid artery
and its progress is visualized if there is blood
circulation. Veith *et al.* (1977) cite the use of
angiography as one source of confirmation of the
validity of the Harvard criteria. But Van Till
(1976) offers angiography as a better alternative
to the Harvard criteria and claims that the Harvard
criteria can leave patients legally open to surgical assault such as organ removal and biomedical
experimentation while they may still be capable of
perception or awareness. Angiography has been more
prominent in European developments, whereas the
EEG has been more widely used and studied in North
America.[10]

One aspect that needs to be clearly appreciated
is the evolutionary character of the diagnostic
criteria. Before the use of ventilators, the clini-

cal criteria were adequate to the needs of physicians. Since that time, however, the EEG has proved
increasingly useful. Hence, the newer criteria
utilizing the EEG can be used as a supplement to
the clinical criteria where needed. Similarly,
angiography is a still more decisive indicator that
has been developed. But this technique is more
cumbersome and time-consuming and could possibly,
in some cases, interfere with the health of a patient.[11] Perhaps, then, it is a method that will
not be in use that often, but it may be regarded
as a supplement to the other techniques in cases
in which a highly conclusive diagnosis is desirable
or necessary. These techniques continue to evolve
and the point is well made by Saunders (1974) that
any conception of death that may have legislative
force should not be tied too closely to specific
medical diagnostic criteria of the time.

Black (1978) reports that future work may pro-
ceed in at least two directions: (1) The search
for better diagnostic tests--a group of radiologists
in New York has proposed a bedside test of blood
flow that might make angiography unnecessary and
other investigators are working on a test for en-
zymes indicating dead cells in cerebrospinal fluid
(Black, 1978, p. 9); and (2) the search for other
combinations of criteria besides the Harvard criteria.[12]

A recent study by the National Institute of
Neurologic Diseases and Stroke (NINDS) proposes
five criteria: (1) unresponsiveness, (2) loss of
spontaneous respiration, (3) absence of cephalic
reflexes, (4) isoelectric EEG, and (5) absent cerebral blood flow.[13]

In 1968 the Presbyterian University Hospital of
the University of Pittsburgh proposed a set of criteria for the diagnosis of brain death. Six kinds
of criteria are required for certification of brain
death: (1) absence of hypothermia or central nervous system depressant drugs, (2) no spontaneous
muscular movements, (3) absence of cranial nerve

reflexes and responses, (4) absence of spontaneous
breathing movements for three minutes with partial
pressure of carbon dioxide above 50 torr at end of
test, (5) isoelectric EEG, (6) failure to increase
heart rate by more than five per minute following
1 mg. atropine sulfate intravenous injection. Grenvik et al. (1978) note that the tests for cranial
nerve activity in number 3--which includes fixed
pupils, absent corneal reflexes, unresponsiveness
to painful stimuli, absence of response to airway
stimulation, no eye movement in head turning, and
no response to irrigation of the ear with ice
water--is meant to be an indicator of brain stem
activity and not merely spinal cord activity.

Jastremski et al. (1978) outline a case that
shows how a careful, standardized approach to brain
death criteria is needed. On admission to an out-
lying hospital, an eighteen-year-old male injured
in a motor vehicle accident was found to be uncon-
scious and unresponsive. He remained in this condition for twelve hours, then, at that point, his
parents were told he was brain dead and they gave
permission for kidney removal for transplantation.

When the patient was transferred to the Presbyterian University Hospital for organ donation, blood
and cerebrospinal fluid were draining from both
ears. He did not react to painful stimuli, but did
have small, reactive pupils and exhibited spontaneous facial grimacing and spontaneous breathing.
He was also very hypotensive. After resuscitation
and treatment, his blood pressure increased and he
began to have spontaneous movements of the extremi-
ties. An angiogram was normal. At that point he
began to improve and after two months he was transferred to a rehabilitation center with only slight
impairment of his cognitive functions.

It is clear that this particular case would not
have been declared brain dead by a thorough application of any of the above sets of criteria. The
point is that if the concept of brain death is to

be used, then standardized, widely accepted and
tested criteria should be effectively met.   This
point is especially applicable to smaller hospitals
that may not have large intensive care units.

A set of criteria proposed by the Conference of
the Royal Colleges and Faculties of the United
Kingdom (*Lancet*, 2, 1976, pp. 1069-70) can be summarized as follows: (1) a deeply comatose patient,
and exclusion of hypothermia, depressant drugs, and
metabolic and endocrine disturbances as causes,
(2) the patient being on a ventilator because of
lack of or inadequate spontaneous respiration, (3)
diagnosis of the disorder should make it clear that
the condition is due to irremediable structural
brain damage, (4) absence of brain-stem reflexes
(the list of these reflexes is similar to the NINDS
and Pittsburgh lists), (5) retesting in as short
a period as seems reasonable for the diagnosis.
It is noted that spinal reflexes may persist.   Finally, neither electroencephalography nor angiography
are required.

A possible danger is that if the criteria for
brain death are not formulated precisely and ade-
quately, an arbitrary notion of brain death could
be adopted.   In particular, arbitrary criteria
could be used as an idiosyncratic way of justifying
the withdrawal of support systems.   But what does
it mean to say that a set of criteria is adequate?
One measure of adequacy is the factor of freedom
from false positive finding.   That is, if brain
death means irreversible cessation of all brain
function, then a set of criteria is adequate if
anyone who fulfills the criteria can be shown to
have irreversible cessation of all brain function.

As Black (1978a) shows, there have been two ways
that confirmations of this type of adequacy have
been carried out: (1) to show that there is no
evidence of brainstem or cortical activity and that
no patients who meet the criteria survive despite

intensive therapy, and (2) to demonstrate that the criteria predict widespread brain necrosis at autopsy.

Numerous studies on the subject of number 1 have been made, but it is especially significant here to report some findings of the NINDS Collaborative Study of Cerebral Death. The institute conducted a study of 503 patients in deep coma who were without spontaneous respiration. Nineteen of these met the Harvard criteria if EEG readings were required twenty-four hours apart. One hundred and two would have met the criteria if only one EEG were required and all of these died, as well. Of 189 of the patients that met the NINDS criteria, 187 died within three months--the other two were both drug intoxication cases (excluded from the full criteria as an exception).

Thus, both sets were found completely adequate in regard to number 1, but the NINDS criteria were more inclusive in scope, yet still completely accurate. Black (1978a, p. 344) concludes that the Harvard criteria accurately predict cardiovascular collapse and somatic death within several days despite supportive therapy. But if the criteria are extended to encompass the NINDS criteria, bodily death can be accurately predicted within three months.

The developments in research in area number 2 as reviewed by Black (1978a, pp. 393-95) are not so clear and definitive. One problem is that there is not complete agreement about exactly what constitutes extensive or widespread brain destruction in such studies. In addition, none of the studies that Black reviews is specifically designed to test either the Harvard or the NINDS criteria. The best that Black can conclude (p. 395) is "that widespread brain destruction is found in virtually all cases in which brain-death criteria have been fulfilled."

Terminology

Often the terms 'cerebral death' and 'brain death'
are used interchangeably in the literature, but in
medical terminology, a distinction of usage seems
to be emerging. Korein (1978, p. 7) distinguishes
as follows: Cerebral death is defined as irreversible destruction of both cerebral hemispheres, exclusive of the brain stem and cerebellum. Brain
death--or its equivalent for Korein, *total brain infarction*--is defined as irreversible destruction of
the neuronal contents of the cranial cavity. This
includes the brain stem and cerebellum, as well as
the cerebral hemispheres and all other contents of
the cranium.

This way of drawing the distinction is clear and
helpful and seems consistent with the trend of
emerging usage. But it can be confusing, because
not everyone adheres to it and because it does appear to beg ethical questions to those who take
the position that irreversible destruction of the
cerebral hemispheres should be enough by itself--
excluding the subcortex--to warrant a declaration
of death.

The exponents of this view, among whom Veatch
should probably be included, or anyone who at least
thinks this view is possible, will tend to think
that requiring total brain destruction as a requirement for "brain death" is to adopt a definition
that is too strict. To these persons, it will seem
that such a definition carries with it too much of
a false negative finding, i.e., some who are really
dead will be declared alive. For those persons,
brain death should be equated with cerebral death.
For them, making the distinction as Korein does
above, between brain death and cerebral death, is
a terminological loading of an ethical question.

We have to be careful with our terminology here.
Brain death is a term that, at least for the purposes of this discussion, must be regarded as open

to different proposed definitions. Certainly it is
taken by many, along with Korein, to mean irreversible destruction of the whole brain, including the
brainstem. By this way of defining it, brain death
is distinct from cerebral death. There are those
who might use the term differently and not simply
by mistake or through linguistic perversity, but
because they think the cerebral hemispheres are
the cardinal locus of life or experience and that
'brain death' should be determined by the irreversible disfunction of the cerebral hemispheres alone,
that brainstem reflexes should not be included.

The thing to note here is that our choice of
terminology is not ethically neutral. Certainly,
however, we must be clear when talking about brain
death to distinguish between cerebral death and
total brain death, whatever term one prefers for
these two concepts. Sometimes cerebral death is
called the apallic syndrome, neocortical death, or
a persistent vegetative state. Often, too, the
words 'coma' or 'persistent coma' are used in a
way that is not clear.

Safety and Certainty of Determination

The argument from tutiorism is that if there is
vagueness or doubt, we should be on the safe side.
In church history and theology, tutiorism (from
the Latin *tutior*--safer) is the doctrine that obedi-
ence to the law is always the better and safer way,
but that an opinion of the highest intrinsic probability in favour of liberty may sometimes be followed. One form of the tutiorist argument on brain
death is that since we do not know whether brain
death or circulatory-respiratory death is, in all
respects, everywhere, the completely appropriate
conception of death, we should always lean toward
the direction of the possibility of life if there
is the slightest doubt.

Thus, Jonas (1974, p. 138) argues: "We have
sufficient grounds for suspecting that the artifi-

cially supported condition of the comatose patient
may still be one of life, however reduced--i.e.,
for doubting that, even with the brain function
gone, he is completely dead."

This argument is one we might call *definitional
tutiorism* and proceeds on the premise that we cannot be sure that brain death is always the correct
definitional conception of death so long as the
circulatory-respiratory conception has any plausi-
bility at all. By contrast, the argument from
empirical tutiorism proceeds from the premise that
there may be specific instances in which we are not
sure whether the concept applies. According to
this argument, in cases in which there is doubt
whether brain death has occurred, it is best to
treat a patient as alive.

Notice that in connection with brain death, definitional tutiorism is, in some respects, more
deeply worrisome than empirical tutiorism. Empirical tutiorism might become manageable if medical
developments produce highly precise criteria for
brain death and our judgements are on the safe side.
But definitional tutiorism remains applicable to
every brain dead patient on a respirator, even if
very specific medical diagnostic criteria are developed. Moreover, even if diagnostic criteria are
not completely precise in determining the very in-
stant of death, a certain latitude of applicability
is permissible as long as the latitude allowed is
ethically harmless.

Any set of criteria for determining some state
can result in two forms of error--false positive
finding or false negative finding. In the case of
brain death, we need to be sure that there is no
reasonable possibility of false positive finding,
i.e., declaring someone brain dead who is not. But
we are not so worried about false negative finding,
i.e., treating a brain dead entity as though it
were or could be still alive. The consequences of
false positive finding could be disastrous, as
virtually every commentator has remarked, whereas

the consequences of false negative finding would
not appear to be of as much significance by comparison.

A wedge argument is one that begins with an apparently small initial concession, but then uses
that initial concession to argue for a like concession of greater importance. In any wedge argument
against brain death, one has to be careful which
sort of error is meant, if the possibility of error
is being used as a ground for rejecting the criteria. Much is unknown about the brain and it follows that it is unlikely that a diagnosis of brain
death can narrow the margin of error down to the
temporal precision that one might attain dealing
with a simpler or better known phenomenon. However, one side of error can be eliminated by allowing the other greater scope for occurrence. In
this case, by allowing a certain latitude of false
negative finding which is relatively harmless anyway, we can eliminate any false positive finding
which may be due to the imprecision involved.

In short, it does not follow from any degree of
indeterminacy of application that a criterion must
be unsafe. It is wrong to be cowed by some latitude
of imprecision into throwing up our hands in de-
spair. This form of reasoning is called the wedge
argument, and like the slippery slope argument we
examine in the next part, it needs to be handled
with care. Not every imprecision can be used as
an argument for rejecting a proposed criterion.

Van Till (1975) argues that the Harvard criteria
mistakenly equate the absence of clinically per-
ceptible signs of life with the absence of life itself (p. 17). She claims this equation is illogical
because a patient under resuscitation treatment
who shows no clinical signs of life might still be
alive. She argues that simply because a patient
shows no reactions to stimuli, it need not follow
that he does not feel the stimuli: "[he] may simply
be incapable of reacting to the stimuli in a manner
recognizable to others" (p. 18). This way of pro-

ceeding, she suggests, illogically puts the burden
of proof on the patient.

One might retort that this refutation overlooks
the EEG criterion, but Van Till rejects that, too,
proposing that while the EEG is a reliable indicator of electrical activity in the cortex, it does
not give reliable information about the deeper parts
of the brain. She concludes that the EEG does not
conclusively rule out the existence of a capacity
for perception (Van Till, 1975, p. 18), and, moreover, it does not show that the absence is irreversible. She feels that the EEG, at best, suggests
the presence of death and only angiography can be
a conclusive indicator.

Veatch (1975) is similarly cautious in remarking
that it is an open question whether parts of the
brain may retain some capacity for function even if
there appears to be no responsiveness or receptivity.
Behavioral observations alone he concurs, are not
enough.

Veatch (1975) also recognizes, like Van Till,
that a flat EEG could be present with brain activity
remaining, because the EEG measures only cortical
activity.

The cumulative effects of these doubts and arguments suggest that the Harvard criteria could contain sufficient imprecision to justify some hesita-
tion on grounds of tutiorism, unless these criteria
are supplemented by others, e.g., angiography. Note
that these doubts are purely theoretical, however.
We have already cited the results of the American
EEG Society study of 1974: no exceptions, barring
drug overdose cases. That, of course, does not
mean there could not be exceptions.

We may be tempted to go even further and argue
from these imprecisions to the impossibility of determining brain death. Currie (1978, p. 180)
argues that because in many brain injuries the damage is not precisely determinable, it is impossible
to make a decision of brain death with any certain-

ty. She argues that this uncertainty exists because we do not have precise scientific facts about
the brain: "After all, we are speaking of an area
of the body in which some ten billion neurons are
packed, in some places in densities of one hundred
million to the cubic inch, each neuron connected
with up to sixty thousand others, no two alike.
It is not surprising that precision is impossible."

This argument, I believe contains two fallacies.
First, because there are cases in which a decision
is difficult or impossible, it does not follow
that every case is undecidable. This is a form of
the wedge argument. For example, because cancer
may be difficult to diagnose in some cases, it does
not follow that the diagnostic criteria are worth-
less or that we can never be sure that anyone has
cancer. Also, as Van Till (1976) points out, the
burden of proof in diagnosing brain death must be
on the physicians. If there is doubt, it must be
presumed that the person may still be alive. But
since there can be doubtful cases, it by no means
follows that a safe decision is always impossible
to make, as we saw above.

The second fallacy is the argument that, just
because something is very complex, it follows that
we can't say anything about it with confidence.
Just because the living brain is formidably complex,
it does not follow that we cannot have clear criteria that will definitely tell us when a brain has
been destroyed. For example, if a brain has reached
the stage of liquefaction, we may declare with
great confidence that it is destroyed, complex
organ that it once was. This may be a form of the
ad ignorantiam fallacy. [14] In any case, it is certainly a fallacious inference: just because we
don't know something about X, it does not follow
that we don't know anything about X. One must be
careful in concluding from imprecision or lack of
knowledge. Mere ignorance of whether a statement
is true need not imply knowledge that it is false.

To so argue is to argue, possibly fallaciously,
from ignorance (*ad ignorantiam*).

Nevertheless, as long as there is room for doubt
we are always brought back to a legitimate question
of great importance: How safe are the brain death
criteria? Is there any possibility that a person
declared brain dead could eventually come out of
coma? Studies have confirmed "no exceptions" to
the Harvard criteria, but occasionally cases have
been cited that seem to indicate there may be exceptions. Currie (1978) marshalls thirteen cases
of coma from which the person eventually emerged
but that could have been declared cases of brain
death at the time of the injury. If these cases are
legitimate, then we should reconsider the Harvard
criteria. She puts forward these cases in an attempt to suggest that we do not know "the border-
line between life and death" and, therefore, we
must reject the brain death redefinition.

The documentation she offers is questionable,
however. Most of the cases she describes are taken
from the *New York Times*, not a source that can be
given much credibility as expert medical testimony.
Much of the expert testimony she does give is from
Soviet physicians, whose findings have apparently
been challenged by neurologists from other countries. Many of the cases she gives do not meet the
Harvard criteria, either because a flat EEG reading
was not demonstrated or because they are hypothermia
cases or, possibly, cases in which central nervous
system depressants have been in use.

Most of these cases seem to equate "coma" with
a prolonged period of unresponsiveness, but surely
this sort of coma in no way refutes the Harvard
criteria. The two most apparently persuasive cases
given are six-year-olds with Reye's syndrome. But
again, it is known by physicians that special cau-
tions have to be taken in determining death in
children. Like hypothermia or drug cases, children
are identifiable possible exceptions to the criteria.

Currie (1978, p. 192), however, cites known drug
cases to throw doubt on the reliability of the EEG.
I don't feel this is really fair, because exceptions of this sort are very clearly recognized by
physicians--see Black (1978, p. 6) or the review
of medical criteria in Walton (1978, ch.3)--and
explicitly in the statements of the Harvard, NINDS,
and Pittsburgh criteria.

Perhaps it is enough for our purposes here to
raise the possibility that there could be significant exceptions to the Harvard criteria, even if
the seriousness of the cases and their actual
definitive documentation remains to be weighed.
According to Currie (1978), Kübler-Ross has reported some cases that had isoelectric EEG and all
other signs of clinical death, but who actually
heard the pronouncement of death.

It such cases are even possible, does this mean,
as Currie (1978) argues, that the whole project of
equating death with brain death should be scuttled?
Not by any means. What it might show is a point
already made by Van Till (1975, 1976, and 1976a)
that the EEG should not always be treated as a conclusive indicator of death without angiography.
Currie (1978) does not even mention angiography,
if her arguments do throw some doubt on the complete and conclusive diagnostic safety of the Harvard criteria, it by no means follows, as she
thinks, that they require rejection of the brain
death concept. At best, they simply underline
the importance of continuing to develop precise
criteria and highly reliable techniques for confirmation, like angiography, as a method to be used
in some cases.

These doubts about the conclusiveness of the
EEG have also been somewhat more cautiously pointed
out by physicians.

Walker (1974) indicates that under certain conditions, e.g., intoxication or hypothermia, there
can be a transient coma with flat EEG readings
that may eventually revert to a normal EEG reading

in a shorter or longer period of time (p. 194).
However (p. 196), he claims that the combination
of clinical findings with a twenty-four-hour recon-
firmation of a flat EEG reading is almost always
associated with a moribund brain. However, he men-
tions other techniques being developed, including
angiographic techniques, metabolic techniques, determination of oxygen consumption, and determination of lactic acid in the spinal fluid.

Harp (1974, p. 394) reports that while the conclusions of the Harvard criteria are widely supported in the literature, there have been reports
of survival following a flat EEG reading in drug
overdose cases, in patients with hydrocephalus, and
in another group of patients with isoelectric EEG's
for various periods with catastrophic brain damage. One of these latter cases survived for one-
and-a-half years and another for two years. Harp
also reports that there have been cases of brain
death without EEG silence. He concludes that the
EEG provides "some small amount of false-positive
information as well as a considerable amount of
false-negative information" (p. 394). He believes
that this is the reason other indicators are being
sought and that "the list of tests that might be
used could be expanded almost endlessly" (p. 394).

We can expect controversies about the applicability of the EEG in diagnosing death to continue. In
the meantime, it seems fair to conclude that there
is some room for theoretical doubt that the Harvard
criteria and other EEG-based criteria are as absolutely safe as every critic might like to believe
they are. Remembering our earlier remarks that
only a very high degree of certainty will reassure
a confused and cautious public, it would seem wise
to maintain some reservations about the Harvard
criteria as the final word.[15]

Veith *et al.* (1977) cite as one proof of the
Harvard criteria confirmation of its findings by
angiography. However, what this will no doubt suggest to some is that using angiography as a supple-

mentary technique is a safer and surer method than just using the EEG along with clinical criteria. For these critics, the NINDS criteria will seem better.

The method of angiography combined with clinical criteria seems to leave virtually no room for positive error. If there is no circulation of blood at all in the brain for just a short period, the subsequent self-destructive cycle of blockage, expansion, and cell destruction would seem to be a very highly plausible, conclusive indication of necrosis of the brain. See Walker (1974), Van Till (1976), and Harp (1974) for clinical descriptions of this destructive process.

We conclude that an excellent case can be made for safety of diagnosis if angiography is taken as a supplement to the Harvard criteria, as in the NINDS criteria. In the view of many physicians, angiography is too invasive a test to be used in many cases, but as a supplementary test for occasional use in difficult cases to diagnose, it would reassure those who have doubts about the certainty of EEG diagnosis.

We must remember the review of the history of experimental confirmation given by Black (1978a) in these deliberations, however. The experimental evidence to date supports the one hundred percent certainty of diagnosis of both the Harvard criteria and the NINDS criteria. That doesn't mean that no mistake can be made in using these criteria, to be sure, but it does tilt the burden of proof in the direction of reassurance.

Part Two

A Miscellany of Arguments

In part one we looked at arguments for and against
proposals for establishing medical sets of criteria
for determining brain death and ways of formulating
clear legislative brain death statutes. In part
three, we will evaluate the conceptual respectabil-
ity of brain death as a target concept that the criteria are supposed to be diagnosing. Meanwhile,
there are a number of other ethical arguments of
one sort or another for or against brain death that
do not fit squarely into either the diagnostic or
conceptual categories. In Part Two, we review and
evaluate this middle class of arguments.

Some of these arguments have a form often called
the *slippery slope,* a common item in medical ethics.
This argument, of ancient lineage, was once called
the *heap* (*sorites*) or the *bald man* (*falakros*), and
arises where it is hard to "draw the line" in the
gradual variation of some magnitude or sequence.
An example given by Max Black (*Margins of Precision,* Cornell University Press, Ithaca and London,
1970, p. 3) has three premises.

Every man whose height is four feet is short.

Adding one tenth of an inch to a short man's
height leaves him short.

Every man who is shorter than some short man
is short.

Therefore, every man is short.

31

The choices of height and increments are imma-
terial--any initial height that is clearly short
will do and any small increment will do. Since
the conclusion is false and the argument is de-
ductively valid, at least one premise must be false.
But which? The third seems above suspicion, and
it is pointless to challenge the first premise;
so it is the inductive step, the second premise,
that analysts of the fallacy have concentrated on
studying.

In fact it turns out to be quite difficult to
specify exactly what is wrong with this sort of
argument, so I shall not attempt to do so here. A
recent solution, "Bivalence and the Sorites Para-
dox," John L. King (*American Philosophical Quarter-
ly*, 16, 1979, 17-25), attacks the inductive step
by constructing an appropriate logic of quasi-
inductive conditionals. All we need note for the
present is that in such arguments the inductive
step needs to be handled with great care and circumspection if fallacy is to be avoided.

There is a causal variant of the slippery slope
that is very often deployed in medical ethics. It
runs as follows: If we allow A, that will lead to
B, which will in turn lead to C, and so forth, until X, some disaster, will eventually follow. In
this variant, one must be very careful on two
counts. First, is the arguer claiming that X *will*
happen, or merely that it *could* happen? Second,
has he filled in all the required connecting steps
of the sequence between A and X? That is, we have
to be very careful to see what the alleged counter-
part to the inductive step is when a causal sequence is suggested.

The Practical versus
the Philosphical Arguments

Van Till (1976, p. 15f) declares that it should
be ethically and legally unacceptable to declare

death to achieve practical ends. She classifies
a number of the well-known arguments for brain
death as practical or pragmatic: (1) the argument
from relieving the burden on family, hospital staff,
etc., (2) the argument from organ transplantation
need, (3) the argument from need for legal protection for transplant surgeons.

Many would seem to agree that these "pragmatic"
considerations should be secondary to the concern
of the health of the patient. I would add that
although there is a significant element of truth in
the claim that (1), (2), and (3) share a characteristic that may not unfairly be called "pragmatic",
we should remember that organ transplantation saves
lives. This end is more than merely pragmatic.
The very distinction between pragmatic and philosophical arguments is prejudicial. Organ donation
may be a pragmatic consideration from the point of
view of the donor, but it will not seem to be to
the potential recipient.

Yet this distinction is widely presupposed by
arguments on brain death. Beecher and Dorr (1971)
argue that practical realities should outweigh
philosophical considerations. They write that the
opponents of redefinition "pit a vague philosophical
view against the here and now of needless loss of
uncounted hundred of lives which might be saved or
at least prolonged by the use of the organs from
a body whose brain is dead" (p. 123). This argument seems to me to make the worthwhile point that
organ transplantation saves lives, but it is certainly fallacious if it implies that the need for
organ transplantation should once and for all se-
cure the equation of death with brain death against
all philosophical objections. An analogy should
show why. Possibly a policy of harvesting organs
from unwilling donors near death would save or prolong hundreds of lives, but that would not make it
right!

Beecher and Dorr (1971, p. 123) even suggest,
against the critics of brain death, that there is

something "ominous, sinister, about a philosophy,
a theology, that unquestionably exact lives for the
sake of an ill-defined philosophical principle."
The suggestion would appear to be that since abstract philosophical principles are "ill-defined",
we may safely disregard them altogether where human
life is at issue. This is a very bad argument indeed. Surely the question is one of weighing the
life of the organ donor against the life of the
organ recipient, and an emotional appeal to the
principle of "life at all cost"--notably itself a
sort of philosophical principle--is not going to
solve or even ameliorate the problem. The question is: whose life at what costs? Just as Van
Till neglects the recipient, Beecher and Dorr ne-
glect the donor.

Notice the contradiction. Van Till rejects
"practical" arguments, including the argument from
need of organ transplants, at the outset. Beecher
and Dorr reject any philosophical considerations
that might conflict with "practical" needs. But
we don't need to worry about the contradiction because neither argument is sound.

Another type of argument for or against brain
death is more determinedly ethical in nature. This
is the approach that not equating death with brain
death is morally wrong or right. Many of these
arguments center around the fact that declaration
of death entails loss of personhood which in turn
entails loss of rights as a human being.

While the opponents of brain death tend to see
as disadvantageous the loss of personhood which
would thereby be declared, the supporters of brain
death see this declaration of loss of personhood
as being morally favourable. According to Veith
et al. (1977), not to accept the brain death criterion is an affront to the person or his memory:
"It confuses the person with his corpse and is
morally wrong" (p. 1653). The argument here is an
aggressive one. Not only is it impractical and
obstructive not to declare brain death, and so

forth, but, it is argued, it is a positive moral
error. To the contrary however, the opponent of
brain death feels that such a declaration may show
lack of respect for the (breathing) person. The
proponent feels that not making the declaration
shows lack of respect for what was the person. It
seems that we are caught in a moral culpability
either way.

Here the brain death exponent takes a more positive and aggressive approach by supplementing all
the familiar practical arguments--organ transplantation and social and economic costs--with a positive moral onous. Veith *et al.* (1977) even argue
that this moral factor is the chief reason for
adopting brain death: "The principal reason for
deciding that a person is dead should be based on
a fundamental understanding of the nature of man."
Without a brain, they continue, the residual activities of the organs "do not confer an iota of
human personality" (p. 1653). This argument is
notable not only for its positive character, but
for the fact that it emphasizes the philosophical
over the more practical factors that are so often
stressed. The argument is based on the premise
that enough people can be brought around to the
view that "some capacity to think, to perceive, to
respond, and to regulate and integrate bodily functions is essential to human nature" (p. 1653). Not
everybody will agree on what man's nature is, but
the authors feel that almost everyone will agree
that if none of these functions is present, a person is no longer alive. Are the argument and its
assump tions too optimistic? Yes--as the sequel
will tend to show.

The case of Tucker v Lower (Virginia, 1972)
shows how little the public really understands the
notion of brain death. In this case, in which a
heart transplant removal from Bruce Tucker was undertaken after a conclusion of brain death by EEG, a
suit of wrongful death was advanced by the donor's

brother. At first Judge Compton charged the jury
using the traditional cardiorespiratory notion of
death from *Black's Law Dictionary*: ". . . [death
is] a total stoppage of the circulation of the
blood, and a cessation of the animal and vital functions consequent thereto such as respiration and
pulsation" (4th rev. ed. 1968). In mid-trial, however, Judge Compton redirected the jury, allowing
them to choose between the traditional legal notion
and the element of ". . . the time of complete and
irreversible loss of all function of the brain."
See Converse (1975, p. 424) for the full statement.
The jury at that point found little difficulty in
quickly declaring for the transplant surgeons,
relying apparently on the "brain death" concept.

The interesting point, however, as noted by Converse (1975, p. 429), is that the jury, as evidenced
by their comments, did not appear to really understand the depth of the question or the concept of
brain death itself. For example, one juror stated
that the trial had proved that a man "cannot live
without a functioning brain" (Converse, 1975,
p. 429).

To me this is an illustration of the difficulties
inherent in trying to "educate" the public about
brain death. Where expert testimony and deep-rooted
philosophical conceptions intersect--as, for example, in the parallel of the insanity defence--
getting clear and broad agreement as a basis for
precisely worded legislation may be presumed to be
very difficult and fraught with pitfalls.

Walker (1974) suggests that the neuroscientist
should not assume responsibility for the decision
that the individual as a whole is dead until the
other vital organs have failed. His reason con-
cerns the difficulties of public acceptance of
brain death: "Only if somatic death can be shown
to follow cerebral death as the day the night, will
the concern be alleviated" (p. 200). The quality
of clarity and certainty required for general assur-

ance and public acceptance of brain death is not to
be underestimated.

Slippery Slope Arguments

One plausible argument against equating death with
brain death is that it sets us on a slippery slope
of sanctioning all sorts of possible surgical as-
saults.

Jonas (1974, p. 133) levels the serious allegation that the major motivation behind the definitional effort of the Harvard criteria is that a declaration of brain death expedites the removal of
organs for transplantation. While agreeing that we
should not artificially prolong the life of a brain-
less body, he feels the proper course is to turn
off the respirator and let the "definition of death"
take care of itself. His worry is that by "redefin-
ing," we set ourselves on a slippery slope of dis-
quieting possibilities. According to Jonas (1974,
p. 137) the first step seems innocent enough--keep-
ing the respirator going until the organs are ready
to be removed, then shutting it off before removal.
But then, he adds, why turn the respirator off so
soon? The ventilated cadaver could be used as a
bank for other organs or a plant for manufacturing
biochemical compounds. It could be used as a self-
replenishing blood bank or for surgical and graft-
ing research. Even further, it could be used for
immunological research or testing new drugs. Finally, even medical instruction is included as a
possibility.

Jonas' point is alleged not to be that anyone
is now actually thinking of such things, but that
one can think of them and that the redefinition of
death has removed any reasons not to think of them
(p. 137).

This is a variant of the slippery slope, the
argument that one thing will lead to another until
disastrous consequences are eventually forthcoming.

Slippery slope arguments have to be handled carefully. First, we have to sort out whether the slippery sequence is something that the arguer is saying
can, might, or *will* happen. Some slippery slopes
have this form. There is a sequence A_0, A_1, ...,
A_k such that if A_0 happens, then A_1 will happen;
and if A_1 happens, then A_2 will happen; and so
forth, up to A_k. Now A_k is something we don't want
to happen. But, as the argument shows, if A_0 happens, then, in the end, A_k will happen. Consequently we should not let A_0 happen. This form of slippery slope might be called the sequential slope.
It can misfire in a number of ways. One way is
that the exponent of it might fail to fill in each
of the necessary steps in the sequence, thereby
failing to establish that A_k really will happen if
A_0 does. Another way is that the exponent might
establish that A_k might happen if A_0 happens, but
suggest fallaciously if he has not established it,
that A_k really will happen if A_0 happens. The
fallacy here is a very effective kind of scare tac-
tic by suggestion. One needs to be careful not to
acquiesce too quickly in the inference that if
something might happen, then it will or must.

In Jonas' case he is content to argue that the
unpleasant possibilities he canvasses are merely
possibilities. He says that perhaps the members
of the medical profession are not thinking of these
things, but that he has shown that one *can* think
of them (Jonas, 1974, p. 137). However, one wonders
whether he is being a little coy when overpage
(p. 138) he writes "the permission [redefinition]
implied in theory will be irresistible in practice,
once the definition is installed in official author-
ity." Here he has gone from a modest *can* to a bold
must. Is this move warranted? I am not satisfied
that it is.

First, it is clear that physicians have a strong
interest in harvesting organs that have been perfused by ventilation of a cadaver. But we must re-
call that anyone who has voluntarily donated his or

her organs for transplantation has done so with the
worthwhile purpose of helping to save life. True,
the whole process sounds frightening, but as long
as the cadaver is definitely brain dead and there
is no possibility at all of awareness or consciousness, some of us would like to donate organs under
these conditions. But the question is whether the
pressure of medical interests will inevitably take
us down the slippery slope to the other worrisome
possibilities suggested by Jonas.

My main reason for thinking that Jonas' argument
does not establish these remaining steps of the
slope is that it is quite possible to maintain and
police a policy of respect for the human body apart
from the question of whether the body is alive.
Organs must be transplanted quickly to save lives,
but there is no parallel urgency to supply blood
or hormones so that it is necessary to use ventilated cadavers for either of these purposes. Of
course there could arise such an urgency, perhaps
because of some unforeseen medical development, but
it is hardly likely that we will tolerate such practices unless they are absolutely necessary to save
lives.

If I had a close relative or friend who had donated his or her organs for transplantation and who
had been declared irreversibly brain dead, I would
not want to allow the ventilated body to be kept
around as an ongoing experiment or biochemical
source, but my grounds for this wish should not be
based on a belief that the person is still "alive".
Rather, it seems more due to my belief that we
should respect our bodies and the bodies of others.
A human body should never be treated indecently or
carelessly.

This respect we have for bodies is something that
would scarcely seem to be affected adversely by
equating death with brain death. Consequently, I
fail to see how the slippery slope to the abuses
Jonas postulates is established. True, adoption
of brain death could lead to abuses, but then again

it might not. Jonas is right to be worried about
possible abuses, but wrong to make a direct inference to the rejection of the brain death equation.

It is enough to refute Jonas' slippery slope to
show that it is possible to have and to enforce respect for dead bodies even if that dead body is declared to be no longer a person. And it would seem
that we would wish to treat a ventilated, brain-
dead body with circumspection and respect.

But is it a respect for what was a person or is
that respect an indication that we still feel personhood in some form is still present? This is the
critical question that tests whether or not we can
be strict adherents to the brain death conception
of the death of the person. My point is that no
argument we have encountered so far clearly excludes
the logical possibility of saying both that a brain-
dead ventilated body is dead, i.e., no longer a
person, and that this body should be treated with
great care and respect.

A form of argument inherent in this particular
slippery slope is the following.

Premise 1:   If X is not a person, X does not have
             rights.

Premise 2:   If X does not have rights, we are under
             no obligations or duties with respect
             to the treatment of X.

Conclusion: If X is not a person, we are under no
             obligations or duties with respect to
             the treatment of X.

The first premise may or may not be true, but we
may presume that it is an assumption of the fore-
going discussions that has this role: If it is
true it leads to certain worries, i.e., with some
other assumptions it leads to a slippery slope.
The second premise is also a component in the slippery slope. But to state it flatly, as above, is
to recognize its dubiousness. The fact is that we

are under duties and obligations to the treatment
of things, i.e., nonpersons that according to Premise 1 do not have rights. For example, we are
under obligations to preserve forests and natural
parklands and we have duties toward animals, obligations not to be cruel to them and so forth. The
argument is valid, but the second premise is false.

Even though a brain-dead ventilated body may
not be a person, it does not follow that we are
under no duties or obligations with respect to it.

Bodies, Dead and Alive

It is tempting to carry the refutation of the slippery slope even further by arguing that a brain-
dead ventilated body is a dead person--that is, no
longer a person--but is still in some sense a "live
body." In other words, "live body" is compatible
with "dead person," but "live body" needs to be
complemented by a negation, "dead body."

This view of the matter seems confusing at first,
and, I would suspect, might not be all that easy
to learn to live with. For one thing "live body"
seems to suggest that there is still some element
of personhood around, suggesting, as it does, the
familiar situation of a live person inhabiting his
or her body. Moreover, the implication that once
a person has "passed away," his body can still remain alive is unsettling, to say the least.

Despite the unattractive aspects of this view,
it has found an exponent in Agich (1976) who argues that there is a "seminal ambiguity" in the
term 'body'--the distinction proposed is that between a "dead body or corpse" and a "mere body"
(p. 100). According to Agich, we distinguish between an alive body or person and a corpse. A
corpse is said to be a body which is dead in that
a person no longer lives in it, but it "is not yet
a mere body in that there may be some life--
cellular, tissue life--in it" (Agich, 1976, p. 100).
Both are dead, but a mere body is even less lively.

This argument seems to involve a contradiction
in postulating brain-dead live bodies, but we have
to remember that according to the proposal, 'alive'
or 'dead' mean something different when applied to
persons than they do when applied to bodies. Thus
'X is a live body' does not imply 'X is a live person'. Despite its peculiar aspects, I believe the
proposal is consistent enough. But can its con-
sistency be uproblematically maintained?

The problem with it as a linguistic recommenda-
tion, aside from producing a fertile basis for more
Scottish funereal humour, is that it tends to suggest, despite its disclaimer, that a "live body"
still contains some relic of personhood. Consequently, it may not be too easy to consistently and
persuasively defend brain death as the death of the
person on this basis.

Agich (1976) tries valiantly to defeat the un-
wanted implication that personhood survives brain
death, but he treads a delicate line. He writes:
"Viewed biologically and physiologically, an alive-
body *grades* into a dead body so that a corpse *may*
yet be alive in some minimal sense and so is not a
mere inanimate piece of matter" (p. 100). We cannot infer from this, however, he continues, that the
distinction between a person and a corpse is without justification. A corpse is a body which is not
a person, because it is dead, but there can be life
in such a body.

This proposal seems to me to contain the seeds
for so much confusion and misapprehension that one
hesitates to get involved in it if there is an alternative.

A less problematic route to making the distinction one wants to make is to say that is possible
to medically distinguish between brain death and
biological death. We can say that a ventilated
brain-dead body can be an organism that is biolog-
cally alive, but the open question is whether biological aliveness of the organism must entail that
the person is alive or even somehow still partially

or proximately alive. The brain death exponent
argues not. For him, brain death is death of the
live person. His oponent disagrees, but they can
both agree to a three-way distinction.

| *alive, i.e., normal, living person* | *brain-dead but exhibits biological life* | *brain-dead with no signs of biological life* |

The kernel disagreement can now be located—it turns
on the question of whether an organism in the middle category is, or is not, a person.

   Hirsh (1975) puts the issue in a similar way:
"The rationale of the brain death devotees is based
on the premise that brain death can be diagnosed
with the same certainty with which biological death
can be pronounced. They contend that it is no
longer necessary to await biological death, since
brain death is equally conclusive" (p. 37). Hirsh
however, tends occasionally to lapse into the idiom
of "live bodies" (1975, p. 36): "Although recovery
of consciousness is impossible [in brain death],
there is no doubt that the 'body' is alive." Note
the quotes around "body". Is a "live body" a
"body"? We seem on the point again of distinguish-
ing between live bodies and dead bodies.

   We don't have to go this far, however, provided
we speak instead of the organism of the dead person
possibly still having biological processes that
exhibit cellular and other forms of biological activity. We can still have respect for the vital
processes in the body, even though the person is
dead by virtue of brain death. No mention of "live
bodies" is needed. The major problem with this
way of phrasing the argument now is that it is open
to the charge of missing the point (*ignoratio elen-
chi*). The point, according to the opponent of the
brain death conception, is that a ventilated brain-
dead individual is alive, not merely because there
are some cellular processes or other biological
activities still in process, but because the cardiorespiratory factor is present. It is not biologi-

cal life that is at issue, but cardiorespiratory
life.   The best way out seems to be refuted.
    The refutation is this: Slipping from cardio-
respiratory life to biological life makes the brain
death criterion sound more harmless than it really
is.   Instead of the three-way distinction above, we
should more correctly have a four-way clarification.

alive, i.e., normal	*brain-dead but*
living person	*has pulse and*
	breathing
exhibits some	*no signs*
biological	*of life*
life	

To be sure, this is even a clearer and finer way of
making the necessary discriminations at the level
of medical description of what is actually happen-
ing in an organism, so the refutation is success-
ful.   The brain death exponent should not try to
reassure us about cadavers in the second category
by shifting the argument by bringing in the notions
appropriate to the third category.
    This refutation makes a good point and helps to
clarify the situation, but can the brain death exponent regroup his forces and overcome it, armed
with the more careful subtleties that have been
introduced by his opponent?   Yes, it seems to me
that this option is open to him.   He can argue that
we ought to have respect for the bodies of former
persons in both middle categories because bodies
in both conditions exhibit biological life.   Bodies
in the second category are likely to exhibit an
even greater degree of biological life because the
oxygenation and circulation tend to preserve metabolic processes that would otherwise be less active.
But the basic reason being cited for respect for
bodies in these two cases is that biological life
is present.
    Still, why should biological life be a good rea-
son for respecting a cadaver that has it more than

one that doesn't? This is a good question that
brain death exponents should look to answering.
The question is made more pointed as medical developments tend to indicate that the slippery slope
postulated by Jonas has become a reasonably likely
possibility. Arnold (1977) suggests that brain-dead
but functioning bodies are "attractive resources
for the advancement of medical knowledge" because
their status as no-longer-persons can allow their
consideration to be utilized. This actual suggestion advances the slippery slope from a *could* to a
might and shifts the burden of proof to some extent
in the direction of the brain death exponent. What
concrete policy guidelines can be formulated to cov-
er experimentation with neomorts?

Yet one needs to be careful even here not to
prejudice the issue. As a rebuttal to a too-aggres-
sive use of the slippery slope argument we pointed
out that just because X is no longer a person it
does not follow that we have no obligations or
duties toward X; so here, too, we must make clear
to the brain death exponent who is too quick to
have us infer that because a neomort is no longer
a person, it may be subject to any treatment an
experimenter might care to put to it. The inference is erroneous, but the legitimate worry is that
in the absence of suitable guidelines, unethical
practices would not be barred.

The question is very pointed indeed. A brain-
dead cadaver may not have rights, on the view taken
by the brain death exponent, but doesn't the person
it once was have the right not to have his body mis-
treated? For surely to maintain a brain-dead cadaver in a state of biological activity without
clear and urgent necessity to save the life of another is an unethical practice. Why exactly is it
unethical?

Very briefly, I believe that such a practice
could be unethical because a neomort, even if not a
person, once was a person and still bears a proximity of relationship to the person it was. Although

it may not have the rights of a person, we are obli-
gated to treat it with dignity out of respect for
the person it once was. Let us be clear that I am
not attempting to say the brain death equation can
be proven and that consequently neomorts are not
persons. Rather I am arguing that even under these
presumptions, it need not follow that we can treat
a brain-dead cadaver like any inanimate physical
object. Therefore, if the brain death exponent is
to maintain the defense I have opened up against
the slippery slope, he must turn to an analysis of
the notion of proximity to personhood that is involved in the high degree of biological activity
possible in a brain-dead but cardiorespiratorily
functioning cadaver.

What this proximity to personhood really amounts
to as a clear and rationally justifiable argument
is not easy to specify. One suggestion is the
corporeal association between the cadaver and the
person it once was, the fact that this tangible
stuff once was or held a person. Another resides
in the physiognomic similarity between the cadaver
and the person it once was.

The latter suggestion can be evaluated by considering the following pointed question. Which
would be more disturbing--the mutilation of the
brain-dead cadaver of a person or the mutilation of
a portrait statue of that same person? The question is made pointed by the observation that portrait statues have an association of resemblance
with a person, so much so, indeed, that destruction
of portrait statues is often a severe expression
of hostility to some personage in times of civil
strife and political upheavals. Yet it would seem
to be intuitively true, at least in my opinion,
that the mutilation of the cadaver would be the
more disturbing of these two possibilities. Yet
this could be irrational in at least one way, for
the cadaver is not likely to maintain this resemblance as long as the statue. It seems, therefore,
that the element of physiognomic similarity may

not, by itself, be the most forceful and rational
argument to account for our intuitions in this
matter.

The second suggestion may be closer to the mark,
for the cadaver more than merely resembles the person it once was. It actually was or at least con-
tained that person. But how could we specify exactly what the required relationship of identity
or containment amount to? Clearly they are tempo-
ralized relationships between something that is
now one thing but is now something else, on the assumption of the present discussion, namely that
personhood no longer persists specifically in the
brain-dead cadaver. These are hard questions in
the philosophy of mind and personhood, but the brain
death exponent must answer them if his case is to
be adequate to our intuitions, or else he must
clearly show why our intuitions are in some way irrational or mistaken.

Finally in this section, we should look at a
more abstractly philosophical argument against the
brain death exponent. This interesting argument
against the equation of death with brain death is
that it is based on a philosphical presupposition
of soul-body dualism. For those who do not accept
the presupposition, the equation may also be rejected.

Jonas (1974, p. 139) argues that we should not
deny the extracerebral body its share of the identity of a person. Therefore, the body of even a
comatose person, if it still breathes and pulses,
"must still be considered a residual continuance
of the subject that loved and was loved, and as
such is still entitled to some of the sacrosanctity
accorded to such a subject by the laws of God and
men" (p. 139). The argument is that we should take
the whole organism as a unity. Even if the brain
may be treated in many ways as uniquely important,
it is philosophically questionable to reject all
other aspects of bodily identity.

Several remarks are in order. First, brain
death exponents often speak of *embodied* consciousness or awareness as the criterion and not simply
mental activity in itself, e.g., Veatch (1976) and
Agich (1976). Therefore, Jonas' remark that they
are not considering the whole organism may be partially inaccurate or exaggerated. In fairness,
however, it should be pointed out that if embodied
consciousness is the central concept, then the
brain death theorist is confronted even more point-
edly by the need to show why, on his conception of
a person, we should have respect for bodies.

Second, it is not clear that the brain death
exponent need be tied to the philosophical position
of "soul-body dualism" without alternatives. All
he need be claiming--see Schiffer (1978)--is that
mental activity is a necessary condition of a person being alive, i.e., without it a person is not
alive. Does this imply "soul-body dualism"? It
seems hard to say. Perhaps more needs to be said
about the implications of brain death for the philosophy of mind. Third, what does Jonas mean by a
"residual continuance" of a person? Unless he
shows that the "residual continuance" is a person, the brain death exponent may still be, as we
saw, entitled to his arguments for the sacrosanctity of the body."

We conclude that this type of argument is not
decisive as a refutation of brain death, but it
raises a number of interesting open questions for
medical ethics. I believe it is Murphy's Law that
states that if something can go wrong, it will. At
present, research on cadavers does take place in
clinical trials for new drugs, under FDA regula-
tions. Also at present, immunosuppressant drug
therapy for brain-dead kidney donors is given that
is not meant as therapeutic for the donor, but
rather for the recipient, so I agree that Jonas had
a good point. I just think he and others have carried it too far in some respects.

A Cerebral Slope?

If we make the move from a whole-brain conception
to a cerebral notion, could an interesting variant
of the slippery slope argument be constructed to
the effect that we ought to look for an even more
specific location for mental activity such as the
cerebral cortex? Or could the argument be carried
even a step further to specific areas of the cortex? Or perhaps yet further to specific neurons
in the cortex? Once we have made the step from
the whole brain to the more specific location of
the cerebral hemispheres within the brain, are we
not then committed to further steps towards greater
precision? Why draw the line at the cerebral hemispheres? These are pointed questions.

Capron (1978, p. 356) criticizes Veatch's position by an argument of this sort.

> . . . the proponents of cerebral death must be pre-
> pared to explain why the line they have drawn at a
> particular level of functioning of a particular
> part of the brain is the most defensible line when,
> given the opportunity to draft an entirely new defi-
> nition, others might feel that a higher standard of
> functioning ought to be required before a person is
> considered a "living human being," a level of func-
> tioning that mentally retarded or senile people (or
> those who did not graduate from Harvard Medical
> School or what have you) may not meet.

The argument is an interesting one, and it is not
clear yet how exponents of cerebral death might respond to it; but it is open to them to say something
like this: if developments in brain research do
establish that the location of mental activity can
be narrowed down more precisely than the whole cerebrum, then indeed our conception of death too will
have to be made more precise. However, at present
the cerebrum is the most precise area that can
definitely and clearly be established. Remember

that in any allegation of slippery slope, what *can* happen should always be clearly distinguished from what *will* or *must* happen. Medical developments *could* establish a more precise area, but so far have not. So the cerebrum is in line with present medical knowledge of the location of cognitive activity in the brain.

This reply is still not entirely satisfactory however. It seems equally plausible to say that mental activity of the higher cognitive sort takes place essentially in the cerebral cortex, the thin membranous substance that forms a mantle over the cerebrum. Why include the lobes of the cerebrum under the cortex if the lower parts of the midbrain or the cerebellum and brainstem are excluded?

Perhaps the cerebral death exponent can give an answer based on facts about brain physiology and function, although I am not sure how he might do this. Perhaps, too, he might argue that it is safer to include the whole cerebrum, because there is a possibility of indeterminacy or error. But then, if tutiorism is brought in, why not be even safer and take into account the whole brain?

This slippery slope argument is not a conclusive refutation of the cerebral death concept, but it does put a heavy onus of proof on the cerebral death exponent to back up his argument more fully.

In confirmation of this argument Black (1978a) states that changing the whole-brain requirement to a definition of brain death that comprises the irreversible loss of capacity for human interaction is more likely to lead to the slippery slope of mercy killing that seems to be the source of much public apprehension about brain death. Whole-brain death entails irreversible pathological brain destruction and subsequent inevitable cardiac death, as the research cited by Black (1978a) cumulatively demonstrates. Even with maximum therapy, patients fulfilling the Harvard or NINDS criteria die within a few months at the outside.

The picture is considerably less reassuring with
regard to cerebral death, however. We have no like
assurance by studies that patients with loss of
cerebral function in a persistently vegetative
state will inevitably die in a short period by
cardiac arrest anyway. In fact, the problem is
exacerbated by the fact that they sometimes do not;
and the clinical picture of the destruction in the
apallic syndrome is more gradual and less marked
by massive, rapid, and clearly irreversible destruction.

Therefore, because the case for whole-brain
death admits of clear, well-established, and widely
corroborated criteria, with a clear clinical picture of pathological destruction that irreversibly
and inevitably leads to death in a short time, we
can see how it is much less open to slippery slope
refutations than the case for cerebral death or,
indeed, any other current candidate that focuses
on one specific part or function of the brain.
The whole-brain concept can meet the slippery slope
hesitations squarely, but it is highly questionable
whether the cerebral concept is on the same position
of soundness.

Concepts and Criteria

Again and again, one finds in the literature on
death and dying the admonition always clearly to
separate the *concept* of death and the *criteria* for
death. This warning is emphasized in the remarks
of Dr. Julius Korein in his preface (1978) to the
encyclopedic *Annals of the New York Academy of
Sciences* volume on brain death (vol. 315). Analysis
of the concept is primarily a philosophical question, whereas the development of diagnostic criteria
is a task of medical science and a subject of current medical research.

The two levels are not--I hope--unrelated to
each other, but, nonetheless, it obstructs clear

discussion if we do not clearly separate, at least
in principle, the level of concepts and the level
of criteria. Usually this separation between the
concept of death and criteria for the determination
of death is insisted on at the outset of a clear
discussion of issues of death and dying, as in Kass
(1971). Although, as I have tried to show (1978,
ch. II), we should probably recognize more than
two levels of discussion and take a multileveled
approach if the situation is to be understood more
clearly. Still, there are the two extreme ends of
a spectrum remaining, the level of concepts at one
end and the level of criteria at the other.

A significant problem is posed by the fact that
it is very often unclear in discussions of brain
death whether the notion of brain death is supposed
to be a concept itself or whether the notion is
simply a way of referring to a set of proposed
diagnostic criteria. Brain death is often thought
to be a technical concept of medical science, as
opposed to death *simpliciter,* which is more widely
admitted to be largely a philosophical notion. On
the other hand, the fact that brain death is very
often defined as *irreversible* loss of brain function or *irreversible*[16] destruction of the brain
suggests that we are dealing with a general concept
and not just specific diagnostic indicators. Indeed, the multiplicity and development of diagnostic tests and proposed criteria suggest that brain
death is a target concept for these criteria and
should not be strictly identified with the criteria
themselves.

Roelofs (1978, p. 40) argues that brain death is
a criterion, not a concept of death. If death is
an irreversible state, then to say a patient is
dead commits us to a prediction of his indefinite
future state. This is the first premise of his
argument. The second premise is that brain death
is presented in the scientific literature as a condition that can be found to obtain in a particular
patient at a particular time or during a finite

interval of time. Therefore, he concludes, brain
death is not a kind of death, for no description
of a patient's present condition can be equivalent
to the statement that he is dead.

This argument is an interesting and significant
one because it highlights the fuzziness of the
status of brain death and the ambivalence of the
literature on the issue of concepts and criteria in
this regard. It is interesting that Julius Korein,
the editor, has put in a footnote to Roelofs' conclusion that brain death and cerebral death are not
new concepts or definitions of death or even candidates for such roles (p. 40): "This volume is re-
plete with disagreement with this statement, but
the reader must separate *concept* of death and *criteria* for death." And that is surely the point
we should take from Roelofs' argument—that there
is disagreement about the point and it should be
looked at more carefully in future.

What the argument seems to me to suggest is that
we should question the presupposition that brain
death is a condition which is said to obtain in a
particular patient at a particular time if we wish
to consistently adhere to the use of the term 'irreversible' or some equivalent in characterizing
brain death.

The best way to approach the matter seems to me
to be to concede that brain death is indeed a concept over and above the particular sets of diagnostic criteria for determination of brain death that
are being proposed. But it seems to be more of a
technical concept of medical science than the concept of death *simpliciter*. The difficulty arises
because brain death is a bridge concept between
the concept of death and the diagnostic criteria
for the determination of death, so it is hard to
know where to locate it in the usual concepts/
criteria dichotomy. But these questions are pur-
sued in more detail in Walton (1978).

Part of the problem here is that there are two
ethical positions to take on brain death which

should be treated as distinct, even if they are
often run together in arguments. One position is
that there is one single concept of death and two
types of criteria for determining when that concept
obtains in a particular case. First, there are the
traditional clinical criteria used in the majority
of cases in medical practice. Second, there are
the brain death criteria for use in the intensive-
care ward, where the use of sophisticated technology makes the use of the clinical criteria inappli-
cable. Here, we have one single concept, but
two kinds of criteria.

The other position is that death is brain death.
That is, according to this second position, death
is equivalent to brain death, so the critical indicator of life is whether or not the brain can function. Then the traditional clinical criteria are
seen as indicators of brain death that may be used
outside special care contexts where failure of the
cardiorespiratory system must shortly be inevitably
followed by brain death (with the usual exceptions
of hypothermia and drug overdose cases).

From the point of view of the medical practice
of determining death, it may not seem to matter
which position is taken, but philosophically, there
is a big difference between the two. The first
position tends to leave the question of what death
is--at the philosophical level--pretty much as open
as it has been. The second position identifies the
death of the person with the death of the brain
and, therefore, singles out this one organ as a
critical locus of the life of the person. It is in
this identification that critics find objections
that a brain-body dualism is presupposed or that
the mind is--questionably--being identified with
the brain.

If you take the second position, brain death
appears to be a general concept of great philosophical significance. Indeed it is equivalent to the
concept of death itself. But if you take the first

position, "brain death" need be no more than a name for a certain class of brain-oriented diagnostic criteria, and these criteria may or may not have much impact on how one philosophically approaches the analysis of the concept of death.

In practice it is often hard to separate the two positions, as they may be subtly combined. For example, Korein (1978) seems to take the first position initially, arguing that brain death criteria are a new development and do not supplant the traditional criteria except in special cases. But then he suggests that the traditional criteria really implicitly were based on a brain-oriented conception after all, because brain death inevitably follows cardiac arrest or extended cessation of respiration. So he appears to make a move from the first to the second position in the course of the development of his argument.

The two positions may be combined, but in order to get a grip on the philosophical basis of the arguments on the issue, it is useful to sort out the two positions in theory. An interesting question is whether the legislative attempts to formulate statutes on death take the first or second position. We make a few brief comments on this question in closing this part.

It seems that some attempts are most likely interpretable as operating on the basis of the second position. For example, the Law Reform Commission of Canada proposal rules that a person is dead when "an irreversible cessation of all that person's brain function has occurred" (1979) and adds that cessation of brain function can be determined by the prolonged absence of cardiorespiratory functions. What this seems to say is that whatever criteria are used, the essential factor they indicate is irreversible cessation of brain function. This is the second position. The ABA model is similar in this regard.

The proposal of Capron and Kass (1972) states that a person is to be considered dead if there is

irreversible cessation of cardiorespiratory function, but in cases of artificial means of support,
the judgement should be based on irreversible cessation of brain function. This appears to be an
instance of the first position. It sets out the
two criteria, but nowhere implies the primacy of
brain function as the concept to be determined.
We just have two different kinds of criteria for
two different kinds of situations.

The Kansas statute is often interpreted to postulate a conceptual dualism that is a "sin against
public psychology" (Law Reform Commission, 1979,
p. 43), but I don't see why it couldn't be interpreted the second way as well.

Perhaps it would be useful to state generally
what counts as a concept and what counts as a set
of criteria, but I shall not embark on such an abstract inquiry here.

Part Three

Concepts of Death
and Brain Death

At last we turn to the more abstract philosophical
arguments for and against brain death that pertain
to the definition or redefinition of death itself.
As we noted, the arguments concerning definitional
tutiorism are, in some ways, more deeply worrisome
and confusing even than the empirical and more
purely medical questions. Here the question is
whether a brain-oriented conception of death as
cessation of mental activity--or whatever notion
one selects from the possible variants outlined,
e.g., in Veatch (1975)--can be established as phil-
sophical prior to a cardiorespiratory conception.

The Cardiorespiratory Conception

It seems reasonable to presume that not too many
educated people today would want to persist in taking the cardiorespiratory conception of death as
exclusively the correct one or even the primary
one. As Skegg (1974, p. 138) suggests, the view of
death as permanent cessation of respiration or circulation is intuitively inadequate if applied to
someone whose respiration and circulation have
ceased, but who is still capable of returning to
consciousness. Such a case need not be purely
hypothetical. The cardiorespiratory diagnosis of
death may be challenged in regard to its continuing universal applicability by the fact that during

certain operations like open heart surgery the body
is cooled and the respiration and heartbeat of the
patient may be stopped for a prolonged period.
Rather the more interesting question is whether
there is still any room for the cardiorespiratory
conception at all. The most significant choice is
between a dual conception of death which combines
cardiorespiratory death with brain death--where,
perhaps, the latter may even be regarded as pri-
mary--and an acceptance of brain death as the exclusive and single conception. It is this dualism
of alternatives that the literature dominantly
reflects and that shapes the current controversies.

One form of argument to weigh the conceptual ap-
propriateness of a cardiorespiratory as opposed to
a brain-oriented conception of death is to imagine
a hypothetical situation in which one is absent and
the other is present. Then we could compare this
with the reverse situation, in which the one is
present and the other absent. Next we could try to
determine which alternative seems more characteristic of death.
    Schiffer (1978, p. 27) poses a pair of cases of
exactly this sort.

Case A. A person X at time t_1 has the following
properties at time t_2 in the operating room: (1)
Cardiorespiratory functions are provided in their
entirety by extracorporeal pump and oxygenator.
(2) The last closure sutures are being inserted in
a massive, posterior, midline incision from occipi-
tal pole to sacrum. Through this incision the entire central nervous system has been removed in
pieces and sent to Anatomy for medical student use.
No upper motor, association, or preganglionic neurons remain with X; X is completely flaccid and
limp; pupils fixed and dilated; no spontaneous
movement or reflex of any sort; flat EEG; no response to any stimulation. Case B. A person X
at time t_1 has the following properties at time t_2:

(1) No respiratory movements discernible over a prolonged period of time by any of the usual, observational procedures. (2) No cardiac pulsations can be identified. There is no apical impulse; no radial pulse, no asculatory evidence of vascular flow. (3) Despite properties 1 and 2, **X shows** clear evidence of a continuing, responsive consciousness. When addressed, X slowly rolls his eyes toward the speaker, moves his lips just perceptibly, and emits appropriate replies in a voice which seems to come from deep within. He also conveys sensation reports, concerning feelings of coldness, and of pain when his legs are tested with a pin.

According to Schiffer, reflection on this pair of possible situations will show that the cardiorespiratory death concept fails at the conceptual level. Case A shows that absence of cardiorespiratory function is not necessary for death, and Case B shows that absence of cardiorespiratory function is not sufficient for death. The other side of the argument is that the brain-oriented (central nervous system) conception of death is not open to the difficulties posed by A and B. Schiffer concludes that the cardiorespiratory conception fails in a way that the central nervous system conception does not.

One thing to notice about this argument is that there is a subtle shift from the brain to the central nervous system as the locus of significance. We return to this question of location of specific physical areas in the last section. There we will see an argument for excluding the spinal cord but including the whole brain. This point aside, is the argument by thought-experiment a good one?

I tend to think it is, up to a point. Some readers may mistrust abstract thought-experiments. And Case B given by Schiffer may not be physically possible. But where philosophical conceptions are at issue, it seems a perfectly appropriate method to adopt. True, the thought-experiment may not be re-

garded as a knockdown argument against the cardiorespiratory conception by everyone, but it does
offer positive evidence to show the thoughtful person that the brain death conception tends to have
greater primacy.

The cardiorespiratory without the brain-oriented
conception is not sufficient for death. It seems
plausible to me that many participants in the
thought-experiment might agree on that much, given
Case B or some equivalent. But is the brain-oriented
conception without cardiorespiratory function sufficient for death? Schiffer seems to think Case A
shows this and, perhaps for many of us, it does,
but I doubt that a hard-liner like Jonas or Currie
would be convinced. They would seem to want to
say that this individual could still be partly
alive. This takes us back to the previous cycle of
argumentation however. If we can have respect for
brain-dead bodies even if we regard them as dead,
perhaps some of the need to worry that A might be
alive can be dissipated.

Thus the best we can say here is that Schiffer's
thought-experiment might, at least for the thoughtful person who finds it plausible, shift the burden
of proof somewhat further in the direction of the
opponent of brain death.

An interesting variant on the thought-experiment
argument is offered by Korein (1978, p. 27). This
version of the argument, however, is not based on
a hypothetical comparison, but on experimental and
clinical cases that exist or could be actually carried out.

Case 1: "If a dog's head is experimentally
severed from the body and kept alive by an appropriate life-support system and the same is done to a
dog's body, the essence of the animal's "personality" is in the head, not the corpus. The head in
such an experiment will eat, salivate, blink, sleep
and respond to stimuli to which it has previously
been conditioned, such as its name being called."
Actual experiments on perfused monkey heads carried

out by White *et al.* (1971) have confirmed these findings experimentally.

Here is an actual comparison case that is so simple and intuitively forceful that it is hard to deny it some weight in shifting the burden of proof. The experiment is a gruesome one, not without its repulsive aspect, but if you think about it, the conclusion that the essence of the animal's personality is in the head is hard to resist.

Ethically, it is not the most favourable case because one's intuitions about where the "personality" resides are complicated by the fact that the subject is an animal rather than a person. But Korein finds an analogous clinical case that even overcomes that problem.

Case 2:   "If a human is quadriplegic because of a cervical spinal cord transection, but has a normal brain, he may be kept alive by a life-support system; unquestionably he is a person who is aware and responds appropriately to external stimuli. However, if a person's cerebral hemispheres were destroyed by a shotgun blast, with subsequent deterioration of the brain stem, the temporary maintenance of his body by modern scientific methods does not mean that a human life is being maintained" (Korein, 1978, p. 28).

This argument is a forceful one because the contrast is powerful, based on actual human cases that could be observed. It is clear that we must treat the quadriplegic as a person. In the gunshot wound case, by contrast, there would be no evidence of personality or awareness at all. True, some reflexes would remain that could create a semblance of life, especially to an observer who is not familiar with the physiology of the situation.

Perhaps as a counter-argument the cardiorespiratory exponent might cite experiments with decerebrate cats that show that spinal reflexes, e.g., some motor reflexes and even sexual responses, remain when the animal has no brain. Could such reflexes be enough of an indicator of life to make

them an ethical factor to be reckoned with in determining death? I can't help thinking that the
more determined exponents of the cardiorespiratory
conception will still see it that way.

Are these remaining motor reflexes any indication of conscious awareness or feeling? The medical experts I have talked with assure me that they
are not, provided the entire brain, including the
brain stem, is destroyed. If such assurances are
correct, then Case 2 does score a telling point
against the cardiorespiratory exponent, for the
presence of these reflexes seem, indeed, to be no
more than a *semblance* of life. It may be a semblance that has a powerful emotional force to a
loved one of the deceased, but, intellectually,
perhaps it is a force that should be resisted.

To summarize, the two cases marshalled by Korein
have to be seriously taken into account in weighing the factors for and against the brain death
equation. Combined with Schiffer's thought-experiment, they represent an argument that cumulatively
interlocks with the other sub-arguments for the
brain death exponent's view to produce a buttressed
position that cannot be easy to refute.

Spontaneity

Veith *et al.* (1977) argue that spontaneous respiration is an indicator of life (p. 1653), but that
it cannot be a definition "since a respiratory patient whose whole defect is paralysis of the motor
neurons to the muscles of respiration due to neurologic disease is surely fully alive despite his
inability to breath spontaneously." Therefore,
they conclude, a loss of respiration must be combined with other evidence, i.e., brain death. This
may be a *non sequitur.* Because absence of *spontaneous* respiration is not sufficient for death, it
does not follow that loss of respiration cannot be
a sufficient indicator. According to Schiffer

(1978, p. 27), it is not spontaneity that is the
essential feature, but rather the flow of vital
fluids itself, respiratory or circulatory, whether
spontaneous or induced.

I would back Schiffer in this, insofar as the
key question is whether an artificially ventilated
but brain-dead patient is still alive. Spontaneity
does not seem to be the main issue. Veith *et al.*
(1977, p. 1654) note that brain death, if it includes destruction of the brain stem, is incompatible with spontaneous respiration. Thus, they
suggest that brain death is simply "professional
jargon" to describe a patient who exhibits permanent loss of signs of life. This includes permanent loss of spontaneous respiration and recognition of it should facilitate society's acceptance
of the concept of brain death and gain public support for legislation (p. 1654).

I am worried here that this emphasis on absence
of spontaneous respiration could be a red herring.
The real point that we should be concerned about
is whether there is respiration, spontaneous or
artificial. True, brain death results in cessation of respiration, but only if a ventilator is
not in use. If the respiration were not artificially possible there would be no problem and this
reassurance would be appropriate. But what we
really need to be reassured about is whether life
in some form could still be present if cardiorespiratory circulation is present, even if brain
death has occurred. This argument does not provide it.

It is interesting to see that the position that
spontaneous cardiorespiratory function is the indicator of life is quite compatible with acceptance
of the position that destruction of the whole brain
is a conclusive indicator of death.

Spontaneity of cardiorespiratory functions has
sometimes been taken as the important factor, for
example by Schwager (1978), who cites with approval
the claim he attributes to Ramsey that spontaneous

heart function is a sign of life. Schwager argues
that this position is in no way inconsistent with
his view that an individual with no capacity for
cerebral function--though he seems to mean by this
the destruction of the whole brain and not just the
cerebrum--may be treated as dead (p. 42). His
reason is that he believes that an individual with
no capacity for brain function cannot have truly
spontaneous heart function (p. 42). This premise
is, however, belied by the statement of Black (1978,
p. 5)--a neurosurgeon--that the brain is not necessary for heart action, at least for many days. According to Black, breathing and heartbeat are different in this respect. If the brain stem is destroyed, breathing ceases, whereas "unlike breathing muscles, heart muscle is so arranged that its
rhythmic contraction continues as long as it has
adequate oxygen and fluid to bathe in" (p. 5). Of
course, if breathing stops, the heart will stop,
too, for lack of oxygen. In that sense, continued
heart function in a properly brain-dead patient may
not be "truly" spontaneous, but it can be, in another sense, spontaneous if blood and oxygen are
supplied.

On the other hand, if Schwager is right that
brain death is not compatible with continued spontaneous cardiorespiratory function, spontaneity is
uninteresting as a factor of serious ethical im-
port, for each and every brain-dead patient, it follows, must be dead by the criterion of spontaneous
cardiorespiratory activity. From this perspective,
brain death--as death of the whole brain--is perfectly acceptable. However, the worrisome problem
of whether ventilated brain-dead patients are still
in some sense alive still remains.

Philosophical Analysis of Death

One way to pose the question "What is death?" is to
ask what features are characteristic of a *person,*

if death may be presumed to be characterized as the
irreversible cessation of personhood. Van Till
(1976a, p. 815) utilizes a doctrine of personhood
to argue for brain death as equivalent to death of
the person. Like Veatch, she likes the word 'inte-
grated' and suggests that a person is, at least, an
organism that functions as an autonomous and inte-
grated entity. A person, she goes on, is more than
a mere living organism. What makes a human organism
into a person is "mental activity" (Van Till, 1976a,
p. 815). She adds that mental activity need not
require interpersonal communication, for there is
no proof that severe mental defectives, newborn
infants, or patients in coma do not have mental activity even though there may be no sign of percep-
tible output.

Most of us might tend to agree that "mental activity" is highly central to a person--whatever
that term might exactly comprise--but, as before,
the problem is that it seems arbitrary to exclude
bodily activity as a characteristic that is also
relevant to personhood. Indeed, I would like to
suggest that a too-thorough preoccupation with the
question 'What is a person?'--a question that virtually comprises the entire subject-matter of the
humanities and social sciences--may be taking us
to some extent away from the point. If death is
the irreversible termination of personhood--the
limit of life--we should be asking not "What is
human life?" but "What is characteristic of the
ending of a human life?"

Until we have a philosophical analysis of the
concept of the death of a person, all the arguments
for and against brain death can, at best, be partial and provisional. Moreover, the specifically
philosophical arguments must remain open if the
target of diagnosis 'death' remains understood
only at a preanalytic level.

Van Till (1975, 1976, and 1976a) characterizes
death as the permanent disintegration of the psy-
chosomatic entity. She argues that this disinte-

gration takes place when and only when brain death
occurs. Therefore, for Van Till, death is equivalent to brain death, where this refers to the permanent destruction of the whole brain. This equiva-
lence characterizes the general pattern of the
arguments for the brain death conception. Brain
death is said to be both necessary and sufficient
for death. We now have achieved some idea of what
brain death means, but, by comparison, the other
side of the equation remains a blank.

Veatch (1976) offers a "formal" definition of
death as "the loss of what is essentially significant to the nature of man." The apparent porous-
ness of this definitional stencil signals that it
is compatible with numerous different analyses or
conceptions of death, depending on what you think
is significant.

Philosophically, it seems that the issue must
remain open until the point at which the candidates
for a concept of death are clearly enough articu-
lated as philosophical models to be evaluated as
components of the brain death equation.

Veatch (1975 and 1976) evaluates a number of
candidates for a philosophical concept of death.
The concept of the irreversible stopping of the
flow of vital body fluids strikes Veatch as im-
plausible. The soul as an independent nonphysical
entity is rejected (Veatch, 1976, p. 42) as "a
relic from the era of dichotomized anthropologies."
Veatch finds the concept of death as the irreversible loss of capacity for bodily integration a more
plausible candidate than either of the preceding
two, but he suspects (p. 42) that it is more attractive because it includes "higher functions which we
normally take to be more central--consciousness,
the ability to think and feel and relate to others."
Veatch then sorts out these so-called higher functions, indicating a preference for some over others.

The criterion of rationality would exclude infants, so it could not be acceptable. Capacity for

rationality would be a criterion that excludes some
senile or mentally incompetent individuals, so it
too must be rejected.

The notion of bare consciousness would include
these individuals, but Veatch rejects it (p. 41)
because he feels it is too individualistic--it
describes a person's life without any reference to
other human beings.

In the end, Veatch's candidate of preference for
a concept of death is "the irreversible loss of the
embodied capacity for social interaction." He thinks
embodiment important and suggests that because of
the requirement of embodiment, we might want to reject as murder the erasing of a magnetic tape that
contains the electrical impulses of a human brain.

My main objection to Veatch's proposal is that
someone might still have the capacity for perception or consciousness even if he has irreversibly
lost the capacity for social interaction. As long
as such a person might be aware of what is happen-
ing, we must surely not treat him as a cadaver from
which organs may be harvested. Indeed, I would
think that any proposed concept of death that al-
lows such a possibility ought to be rejected out-
right for that reason alone.

Another objection I have is that consciousness
should not be rejected as a criterion even if it
could, as Veatch suggests, be described without
reference to any other human beings. I am sure
we applaud the notion that man is a social being,
but I do not believe this premise is a good basis
for concluding that a person who has lost the ability to communicate socially may be declared dead.
As Van Till (1975, p. 140) rightly insists, it is
most important that a patient not be declared dead
if there is even the smallest possibility that he
can feel pain or hear his future discussed. Surely
Van Till (1975, p. 137) is right that if there is
the possibility of perception, there should not be
any basis for declaring death. The fundamental
question is whether the individual retains the

faculty to be aware or not. True, this faculty en-
ables communication and social interaction, but the
point is that it could be present without social
interaction.[17] Thus, the capacity for social interaction criterion must be ruled out on grounds of
tutiorism.

Some commentators prefer 'perception' as the
primary indicator. The problem I have with this
term is that it seems to emphasize the sensory faculties at the expense of the higher cognitive element of reflective consciousness. According to
Van Till (1975, p. 136) the criterion of death
should be the faculty of perception--it is not,
she rightly insists, a question of how well perception functions, but whether there is perception at
all. Since perception can possibly exist if the
synapses and neurons of the brain are still functional, she argues that only a conclusive demon-
stration of brain death by angiography is sufficient
to declare death and allow possible organ transplantation.

This position raises the question of what is
meant by "perception." Van Till (1975, p. 137)
says that two-way communication is not essential--
receiving and processing information is enough.
This suggests an ambiguity however-- 'perception'
is sometimes meant to denote the reception of information, but sometimes also covers its processing
or recognition. I would prefer the word 'consciousness' because a person might not have the ability
to perceive--in the sense of reception of informa-
tion--but might still be alive if consciousness persists. Moreover, the term 'perception' might apply
to reflex actions, e.g., blinking, which might not
indicate conscious awareness. But 'perception' is
not unsatisfactory if this term is understood in a
broad fashion.

The pupillary reflex is mediated through the
lower brain stem, so Van Till would have to include
the presence of this reflex as a possible indicator
of life, since she requires destruction of the whole

brain to be demonstrated for a declaration of
death. However, Veatch (1975, p. 24) excludes
pupillary and withdrawal reflexes on the ground that
the ability to maintain nerve circuitry to carry
out these reflexes "does not really add significantly to man's integrating capacity." At other
times, however, Veatch (1975, p. 29) claims that
the central concept is that of experiential and
social functioning. Once again, one senses that
the terms 'experience' or 'perception' tend to be
used ambiguously. Or perhaps it is partly a physiological disagreement. Veatch (personal correspondence) fails to see how the presence of a pupillary reflex indicates any capacity for perception
and how it could indicate a possible presence of
life, but I don't feel that we can talk of such
matters in a way that suggests that the issue is
established in any black-or-white way. The pupillary reflex could, for all we know, indicate some
presence of feeling or sensation even if the higher
cognitive faculties are absent. Even if we cannot
resolve the issue with the precision we would like
and, indeed, just because of that, we should be on
the safe side.

Michael Newman concedes (personal correspondence) that loss of mental activity is a major dimin-
ishment of life, but even when this is lost a person may still be able to feel pain or pleasure. He
distinguishes between perceptions which indicate
some cognitive function and sensations which require
little if any; but when all sensory activity is
gone, then he feels that anyone would agree that we
are left with vegetative existence and that the patient is dead.

Following my tutiorist line of argument, it is
clear that we cannot rule out the possibility that
brain-stem reflexes could indicate some form of sensation of feeling, even if higher mental activity
is not present.

So far in this section we have concentrated on
conceptions that take one feature as primary or ex-

clusive. What about a more pluralistic approach?
The philosophical possibility of viewing death as
a dual concept--containing elements of both the
brain and cardiorespiratory concepts--has been said
to be implied in the legislative proposal of the
Kansas statute (1970). This statute, we remember,
states that a person will be considered dead if
there is absence of spontaneous respiration and
cardiac function or if resuscitation is considered
hopeless. A person will also be considered dead
if there is an absence of spontaneous brain function. One of the most serious criticisms of this
statute we discussed above is its apparent implication that a person could be dead in one sense, but
still alive in another sense. This sort of ambivalence is hard to tolerate philosophically and, perhaps, even harder to get the general public to
understand or appreciate.

Part of the difficulty here, as we have already
mentioned, is a confusion between concepts and criteria. It seems tolerable that we can have a number of different kinds of medical criteria for determining death, based on different contexts of
diagnosis. For example, the clinical criteria may
need to be supplemented by EEG or angiography in
certain circumstances, but it is highly question
able whether we may infer from this that the concept
of death itself is ambiguous. This fallacy is easy
to commit and worth discussing.

Even if we cannot argue straightforwardly from
a plurality of diagnostic criteria to a conceptual
plurality, it is still true that conceptual plurality, whatever its basis, is a bitter pill to swal-
low. The idea that person X could be both dead and
not dead at the same time is highly problematic,
ethically and conceptually, not to mention its general acceptability to the public. Here is a view
that is only worth trying to defend if all reasonable alternatives are definitively ruled out.

Yet the establishment of one single element, the
absence of which may reasonably and surely be pre-

sumed to be the characteristic of death, must be
regarded as not accomplished. This *lacuna* in the
argument for brain death must surely be the largest
gap we have found. Still, it must be said that
Veatch, Van Till, and others have made some progress in evaluating the possible alternatives.

Part of the general problem is that, with a few
exceptions, philosophers have not really perceived
the analysis of the concept of death as a subject
for research. True, existential philosophy has
been preoccupied with death as a topic, but that
tradition does not appear to have produced a clear
enough analysis to provide a definite target concept for diagnostic criteria of death. Veatch
(1976) presents several philosophical models of
death; but, again, these models are not developed
in a highly analytical way, and one is struck by
their multiplicity.

The literature in the analytic tradition is not
yet in a mature stage of development. Van Evra
(1971), in a short but provocative article, developed the Wittgensteinian idea that death can be
conceptualized as a *limit*. That is, death should
be thought of not as a positive object of life or
experience, as many existential thinkers have
seemed to imply, but as a limit or boundary of life.
Just as the limit of my visual field cannot be itself within my visual field--or it would not be the
limit--so death cannot be itself within the life-
experience. Rather death is like a function that
orders the members of a series that are limited by
it. This view is highly reminiscent of the Epi-
curean tradition that death is not itself an item
of experience to the *moriturus*.

Nagel (1970) criticized this sort of view as
inadequate to our language of possible but non-
actual alternatives when speaking of death. Do we
not often say that a person's death is tragic because of what he could have been or could have done?
If so, does this not commit us to talk of possible
alternatives and possible--but nonactual--persons

as the subjects of these possible alternatives?
True, the view of death as limit relieves us of the
need to postulate "experienceless selves," and some
would say that is an advantage. But how can we make
sense of statements about what could have been or
might have been, had it not been for death, if it
makes no sense to talk of persons other than in
terms of categorical states in the life of an individual?

To work toward an adequate and unified account
of the concept of the death of a person, I introduced (1978) the dual theory of death both as the
limit of life and as the superlimiting notion of
a possible person. According to this view, death
is the limit of life, but it is also necessary to
understand death in terms of possible alternatives
that transcend the limit. Death so understood, I
have argued, is even compatible with the secular
belief that the actual person is completely destroyed in his death and ceases to exist as an
(actual) person.

The view of death as limit is a comparatively
safe view, sure to be favoured by empiricists, who
tend to regard possible persons of any sort as sus-
picious characters. Moreover, as Woods (1978) has
shown, talk of possible persons is characterized
by numerous conceptual difficulties that make it
a hard bit of language to understand clearly. On
the other hand, as Woods convincingly shows, the
view of death as superlimit is essential if we are
to make sense of most ordinary statements about
death, often comprising as they do, potentialities
and possibilities.

Do any of the developments sketched above relate
to the question of brain death? I think they do,
in the following ways. If death is the limit of
life, the limit or boundary in question is not the
cessation of functioning of any physical process
in the body like respiration or circulation of the
blood. It is the limit of conscious awareness, of
experience, and of thinking. Medicine, biology,

and related sciences tell us that the brain is the
locus of conscious awareness. Therefore, it is
natural to identify death with brain death.

If death is viewed as superlimiting possible alternatives projected beyond the limit, one natural
way to look at such possible alternatives could be
as mental constructs, scenarios that represent re-
constructions of what might have been. We are speaking of objects of thought, and therefore again the
language is that of conscious processes of thought.

Some might say that this dual viewpoint does not
make death out to be enough of a physical process,
an actual event in the history of an organism. But
we should remember that we are adhering to a distinction between concepts and criteria. The abstract concept of death, to be implemented in practice, does need to be correlated with physiological
criteria. Once it is, the physical aspect of the
concept is restored.

Which Areas of the Brain?

Is it the destruction of the whole brain or merely
the cortex that is significant? The EEG measures
cortical activity, whereas angiography is a determi-
ner of whole brain death, so we could expect a
division of opinions here. It is also a matter of
philosophical preferences. Van Till likes the criterion of total, conclusive, and irreversible absence of all perception; and, therefore, she is in-
clined toward the whole brain idea--and, consequently, angiography. Veatch (1975) sees as persuasive the argument for the centrality of "experiential and social functioning" and, therefore,
favours neocortically oriented indicators .

According to Van Till (1976a, p. 815), neurologists disagree as to the precise location in the
brain of the function she calls mental activity.
Some cite the cerebrum, whereas others propose the

whole brain. Thus, she cites *Dorland's Medical
Dictionary* as suggesting that we should clearly
distinguish between brain death and cerebral death.
Korein (1978) also makes clear the necessity for
appreciating this distinction, as we remarked in
part one. Throughout, we have seen arguments that,
to be on the safe side, we should presume that the
whole brain is required to produce mental activity,
and not merely the cerebrum or some other part.

This argument from tutiorism seems sensible.
Why exclude the brain stem or other parts of the
subcortex, if there is a possibility that some element of consciousness could remain in an individual
with destroyed cortex or cerebrum, but with other
areas intact? As before, we argue that vagueness
is permissible as long as the possibility of error
is on the safe side. Requiring the destruction of
the whole brain seems to be the only perfectly safe
course, unless biomedical research develops a more
precise location of that characteristic thought to
be central and philosophical research better identifies that characteristic.

One could always retort: Why not be safer and
include more than the brain? Why exclude the spinal
cord if it contains neurons and synapses similar to
those in the brain? Van Till (1967b) has some arguments in reply. She suggests that because the number of neurons and synapses in the spinal cord is
many times smaller than those in the brain and the
nuclei lie further away from each other in the
spinal cord, there is at least a gradual difference
between cord function and brain function (p. 817).
Second, the spinal cord is only accessible to tactile stimuli, whereas the brain is accessible to impulses from all five senses. Third, the output is
different--only the brain can produce mental activity. She claims that this is confirmed by the fact
that patients with a high spinal lesion cannot perceive pain stimuli below the level of the lesion,
but they can sometimes react to such stimuli by
movements.

The upshot is that brain death should include the whole brain but nothing more. I would add that especially if we emphasize the element of reflective selfconsciousness or awareness, as suggested above, the tactile stimuli accessible from the spinal cord need not be thought significant if, in the absence of a brain, there is no possibility of awareness of these stimuli. The presence of a tactile reflex by itself need not indicate mental activity or consciousness.

There is a kind of logic to the position of Veatch (1975) that cerebral death should be preferred to whole-brain death, even though the risk of error may be greater in determining the former with certainty, for if death is the irreversible loss of the higher cognitive faculties of thinking and interacting meaningfully with others, it would seem to be the case that the destruction of the cerebral hemispheres would ensure the loss of these higher capabilities. Therefore, it would seem illogical to say that a patient with cerebral death could still be "alive."

The argument seems sound and commands our attention, but three comments should be made on it. First, one can question the premise that death is the cessation of the higher cognitive faculties. Even though the so-called higher capabilities are absent, remaining vestiges of perception or awareness might still make one wonder whether life could be present in some form. Whether any kind of awareness might still persist while neurons are functioning in the deeper parts of the brain under the cerebrum is a difficult question to answer. Some would want to say that death is the cessation of all perception, whether of the so-called "higher" sort of awareness or not.

Second, although the argument may be sound, it is hard to know how to define exactly what is meant by "higher cognitive faculties," so it is hard to be sure that we mean by this phrase something that

definitely excludes all types of perception that
might persist in the deeper parts of the brain.

Third, as we have seen, it is presently not a
straightforward, definite, and unproblematic matter
to diagnose cerebral death. Consequently, although
the argument may be sound in principle, it is questionable whether cerebral death could be diagnosed
with adequate certainty to preclude the risk of
positive error, so on grounds of tutiorism, the
argument cannot be practically implemented for
ethical reasons.

In an instance of this sort, it may be all right
to do something that may turn out to be "illogical"
or at least inconsistent with certain premises we
have adopted, provided we do not presently know
for sure that we are being "illogical" and that it
is very important to be sure. In cases in which we
do not know for sure, the margin of error may need
to allow for some possible false negative finding
to counter the risk of making a false positive finding.

Veatch (personal correspondence) suggests that
it counts against my tutiorist argument that certain
minimal brain function remains even when the Harvard
criteria and other stringent criteria are met. The
reply is that of course there may be isolated cell
functions of some sort even after total brain infarction. Whole-brain death need not imply the
cessation of even the tiniest bit of cellular or
ionic functioning. The point is that if the whole
brain undergoes the process of destruction and cell
cannibalism characteristic of total brain infarction and the brain stem and all major functions are
included, then there can be no reasonable doubt
whether sensation or awareness persists.

As Korein (1978, p. 6) puts it, ". . . in order
to develop criteria to diagnose brain death, it is
not required that every neuron in the brain be
destroyed. Rather, it implies that the extent of
destruction and consequent irreversible neuronal

dysfunction is so great that regardless of any supportive measures, irreversible cardiac arrest and
death of the adult human being is inevitable within
one week." Thus, if we take into account the limits
of what we do know and what we don't know about
brain destruction and loss of brain function, requiring whole-brain death is not illogical or inaccurate. It is the most rational alternative
available when the ethical requirements of safety
are uppermost.

The term 'apallic syndrome' is another term that
means the same as what Korein (1978) calls cerebral
death--it refers to the loss of the pallium, the
grey cortical mantle that covers the cerebral hemispheres. The apallic syndrome implies a severe
total or almost irreversible destruction of the
cerebral cortex, according to Ingvar et al. (1978)
and its clinical symptoms include the following:
complete loss of higher functions (speech, volun-
tary movement, emotional reaction, signs of memory),
depressed or isoelectric (flat) EEG, low cerebral
blood flow in most cases, and almost total destruction of the cerebral neurons. Brain-stem function
is, however, retained, with the result that there
can be spontaneous breathing and primitive motor
reactions, e.g., swallowing and blinking. Ingvar
et al. (1978) report that the cortex had been replaced by a "thin gliotic and fibrous tissue" in
those patients who had survived in this condition
for several years. Two cases of patients in this
condition are reported by Ingar et al. (1978) to
have survived for eight and seventeen years respec-
tively.

Ingvar and his associates prefer the term 'apallic syndrome' to the term 'cerebral death' (or to
'neocortical death', another term sometimes used)
because of the linguistic similarity of those latter terms to 'brain death'. They note that laymen
and even many doctors do not always appreciate the
difference between the cerebrum and the whole brain

(including the brain stem). The inclusion of the
word 'death', they suggest, appears to add to the
confusion--see Ingvar *et al.* (1978, p. 200f.).

As an illustration, it may be worthwhile sum-
marizing one of eight cases described by Ingvar *et
al.* (1978). The patient was a female who had been
born in 1936. In 1960, at the age of twenty-four,
she suffered a severe epileptic attack during preg-
nancy followed by a deep coma and transient cardiorespiratory failure. Angiography showed signs of
deterioration of the brain. The EEG reading did
not reveal any cerebral electrical activity and
remained isoelectric for the rest of the survival
time--seventeen years. After the first three or
four months, the state of the patient became stable
"with complete absence of all higher functions."

The description of this state is summarized as
follows. The patient lies supine and motionless,
with closed eyes. Spontaneous breathing takes
place through a tracheal cannula (a hole cut in the
throat). The pulse is regular. There is severe
contraction of the limbs--the posture somewhat resembles a fetal position. There are responses to
signals, including eye-opening, movements of the
hands or feet, chewing and swallowing, and withdrawal reflexes. Various eye-reflexes are present.

Measurement of blood flow in the brain indicates
a low average flow in the cerebral hemispheres and
an abnormal distribution of flow, the higher rate
of flow being over the brain stem.

The patient eventually died of heart disease.
The autopsy showed a shrunken brain with atrophied
cerebral hemispheres "transformed into thin-walled
yellow-brown bags." The cerebral cortex was almost
totally destroyed.

It is an interesting question whether patients
in an apallic syndrome should be considered as possible donors for transplantation. Dr. Michael Newman of the Saint Boniface Hospital in Winnipeg has
told me that his policy is not to consider recommen-

dation as a possible donor unless there is total
brain death, including irreversible destruction of
brain-stem function, but to consider the possibility
of withdrawal of treatment in certain cases in which
there is irreversible destruction of brain function, excluding the brain stem.

A similar policy is indicated by Dr. Ingvar of
Sweden in discussion (*Annals of the New York Academy of Sciences,* vol. 315, 1978, p. 210). He suggests that persons in an apallic syndrome must
presently be considered "alive" and should not be
organ donors. His reason is that we do not yet
have enough knowledge of this type of case, nor
have the ethical issues been sufficiently explored.
His cases suggest that it takes some years before
the white matter of the cortex disappears and that
the destruction is progressive. More study, then,
including the use of computerized tomography scan-
ning, could simplify diagnosis.

A question that has not been explicitly asked
about the considerations on brain death is this:
What is meant by the term 'irreversible' when one
characterizes brain death as irreversible destruction of the brain? This term means that brain function *cannot* be restored, that it is in some sense
not *possible* for brain function to be restored.
But what sense of *possible* or *can* is specifically
meant? Presumably, it is not *logical possibility*
that is meant, for there is, we may presume, no
logical contradiction in even a putrified brain's
being restored to functional status. Presumably
some sort of *biological* or *physiological possibility* is meant--a possibility relative to biochemical
laws taken together with facts about the mechanisms
of the neuronal and synaptic structures of the human brain.

One problem is that the notion of possibility involved here is one that has been very difficult, in
numerous other philosophical contexts, to develop a
clear analysis of. Philosophers have disputed in-
tensely over what is meant by the sense of impossi-

bility expressed by statements like "I can't run a
mile in five-and-a-half minutes this morning," and
numerous explanations have advanced; but the problem remains largely unresolved. The meaning of *can*
has played quite a role in ethics, especially in
problems of freedom and determinism.

One might try to get around this difficulty by
avoiding the modality of impossibility and talking
about brain death simply as cessation of brain function. But I think this is not good enough because,
depending on how you describe cessation of function, a brain that has ceased to function could
possibly at some later point begin to function again.

I believe that in this regard the whole-brain
death exponent is on much safer ground than the
arguer who wishes to equate brain death with cerebral death, for it is possible for a person to be
in coma with disfunction of the cerebral cortex due
to injuries when, because of changes in the reticu-
lar formation of the deeper brain, cortical function eventually returns after an indefinite time.
Here there is, indeed, cessation of function of the
cerebral cortex, but it is often very difficult in
such cases to know whether a patient who evidences
such cerebral disfunction exhibits irreversible
brain death. Such a disfunction could be reversible
for all we know, even though the coma might last
a long or indefinite period of time.

However, in total brain infarction, the neuronal
destruction is so complete that medically, there
can be no doubt that the brain has been irreversibly
destroyed. In total brain death, cardiac arrest
ensues within a week or so at the outside--see
Korein (1978, p. 7). In any case, it is clear that
all brain function has disappeared regardless of
what resuscitative measures might be applied.

Concluding Remarks

An interesting argument of Korein (1978, p. 2) is
that both the traditional clinical criteria and

the new brain-death criteria are, as he puts it,
"actually predicated on an implicit *concept* of brain
death." A critic would want to know why the traditional cardiorespiratory criteria must be thought
to be predicated on an implicit concept of brain
death. Why is brain death implicit? Korein's argument is based on the premise that the death of the
brain inevitably follows total circulatory and respiratory failure within a few minutes. He remarks
(1978, p. 2) that it is only in the relatively in-
frequent situation of intensive care that the brain
dies before the other systems being maintained by
technology.

I say that this argument is interesting because,
if it is correct, it would go a long way toward
establishing the equation of death with brain death.
If Korein's argument is correct, there is no need
for a cardiorespiratory conception of death at all.
We have two sets of criteria, the clinical--largely
based on pulse and heartbeat--and the brain-oriented,
and both exemplify the concept of death as brain
death. At the level of concepts there is no multiplicity at all--death is univocally brain death.

Let us look at the argument more closely; it
runs as follows:

> The death of the brain inevitably follows total
> circulatory and respiratory failure in a few min-
> utes. Therefore, the traditional cardiorespiratory
> criteria must be predicated on an implicit concept
> of brain death.

The connection between the premise and conclusion
is not readily apparent. If event B always follows
event A, inevitably in a few minutes, why need it
be the case that A must be predicated on an implicit
concept of B? The inference is by no means uni-
versally valid, it would seem. Mere constant con-
junction of two events A and B would hardly seem to
be sufficient evidence to establish a relationship
of implicit conceptual predication between A and B,

unless one is very much a Humean about what "conceptual predication" amounts to.

Why can we not consistently accept the premise
and deny the conclusion? It seems we can, so the
best that the argument establishes is that cardiorespiratory criteria are at least consistent with
the use of the concept of brain death. Further
premises are needed to establish that cardiorespiratory criteria must involve implicit use of the concept of brain death.

Korein (1978) argues that the brain is the critical system of the human organism because it is the
only system that cannot be replaced by an artifice.
Therefore, if the brain is irreversibly destroyed,
the critical system is destroyed and the organism
as a functioning entity no longer exists.

While I don't dispute the conclusion of this
argument that the brain is, in some sense, the
critical system, I don't like the argument. Because
an organ cannot be replaced by technology, it does
not seem to me to follow necessarily that it must
be a critical system in that its irreversible failure causes the organism as a functioning entity to
cease existing. A pancreas cannot be replaced by
an artifice. It may be true that if your pancreas
is irreversibly destroyed then you will be dead.
But even granted the premise that a pancreas cannot
be replaced by technology, why should it follow
that the pancreas is the critical system so that
its destruction implies the cessation of the existence of the organism as a functioning entity?

Still, there may be something in the argument.
The brain is a critical system insofar as its complete destruction does result in such imbalances
and destruction in the rest of the body that a rapid downward trajectory of the remaining system ensues. Provided the brain stem is destroyed, the
cycle of destruction is rapid and irreversible--
usually a matter of a few days until cardiac arrest--
and supportive measures cannot stop it, but only
postpone it. As Korein (1978, p. 26) puts it, "the

human organism is no longer in a state of minimal
entropy production; its state will progressively
become more disorganized by spontaneous irreversible
fluctuations."

In looking over the arguments for and against
the equation of death and brain death, one is struck
by their open texture, the continually changing aspect of their development, and the inconclusiveness
and *lacunae* of the total network of argumentation.
It would be tempting to conclude that because there
remains much we do not know about the equation it
is false or may be rejected. But to argue thus
would be to once again fall into the ever-tempting
pitfall of the *ad ignorantiam* fallacy. Because the
equation is not known to be true, it does not follow that it is known to be false.

On the other side, it might be tempting to conclude that since none of the refutations of the
equation have definitely succeeded in establishing
its falsification, we may accept it as true. This
is the other side of the same counterfeit coin:
because the equation is not known to be false, it
does not follow that it is known to be true.

Looking over the complex of arguments, perhaps
the best we can fairly and accurately state is that
a solid weight of argument for an initial case has
been made for the equation of the death of the person with whole-brain death. The same case cannot
be made for cerebral death, however. If recent developments are taken into account, the whole-brain
criteria show all indications of safety and the
philosophical proposals for indicators of death
show promise of analytical development. However,
more informed ethical reflections and philosophical analysis would help a great deal.

Some of our most useful findings have been to
expose the weaknesses and *lacunae* in some of the
brain death arguments. We are at least in a position of Socratic wisdom: We now know what it is
that we do not know and what we need to know. Further, because no existing refutation of the whole-

brain concept is conclusive and some positive arguments, however inconclusive in the end, have been
brought forward, we may say that the burden of
proof tilts significantly in favour of the brain
death exponent. This could change, however, and
further research and argument may be expected to
concentrate on the *lacunae* uncovered.

We have seen that whole-brain legislation may
not have the widespread impact some expect, for
we are not talking about patients in this category
who need to be supported in a comatose state for
very long periods. To counteract the notion that
hospitals are filling up with brain-dead patients,
Dr. Ingvar (*Annals of the New York Academy of Sciences,* vol. 315, 1978, p. 208) in a discussion,
noted that the average time of survival is only
three to five days. Thus, total brain death is not
a severe economic problem, whereas the production
of apallic patients by rescusitative care is, in
this regard, more of a problem, because patients
with only cerebral death and an intact brain stem
can survive for several years, in some cases. Dr.
Korein adds in a note that the maximum time to
cardiac standstill in brain-dead adults appears to
be one week (p. 208). More recently, however, Grenvik *et al.* (1978) report that, to the best of their
knowledge, the longest case was that of a young male
reported to be treated in an intensive care unit for
thirty-six days. In this case, brain death was re-
peatedly documented by clinical evaluation and angiography. Grenvik *et al.* (1978, p. 286) note, however, that the usual time to cardiac arrest in
brain death cases is three days.

It is to be hoped, however, that further studies
of the apallic syndrome will give better indications
of how to deal with ethical problems posed by long-
term care of persons in persistent vegetative states.

Notes

1. We use the term 'brain death exponent' to refer to anyone who accepts the equation of brain death with the death of the person.
2. Ontario Natural Death Act, Bill 3, 1977. Printed in *Essence*, 2, 1978.
3. A useful review of the various bills to legislate treatment refusal has been compiled by Dr. Robert Veatch and is available from the Hastings Center.
4. See Converse (1975) for fuller details and discussion. This case has its controversial aspects. Robert Veatch has argued that the jury only determined that Lower was not guilty of the wrongful death of the patient, thus, theoretically leaving open what concept of death they used.
5. For further information see William J. Curran, "The Brain-Death Concept: Judicial Acceptance in Massachusetts," *New England Journal of Medicine,* 298, 1978, 1008-9, and, by the same author, "Settling the Medico-legal Issues Concerning Brain-Death Statutes," *New England Journal of Medicine,* 299, 1978, 31-32.
6. If we identify brain death with cerebral death, perhaps a case could be made for discussing the Quinlan case in terms of brain death, but see the comments on cerebral death in Part Three.
7. Note that 'brain death' as here used is to mean whole-brain death, as contrasted to cerebral death. See the next section for a detailed description of this distinction.
8. See Walton (1978, ch. 3).

9.   See Harp (1974) and Black (1978a) for further
details.
10. See Van Till (1975) or Walton (1976) for details.
11. See Walker (1974).
12. A report of a number of new techniques being
studied experimentally is given by A. Earl Walker,
"Ancillary Studies in the Diagnosis of Brain Death,"
*Brain Death: Interrelated Medical and Social Is-
sues, Annals of the New York Academy of Science,*
315, 1978, 228-40.
13. For fuller details, see Black (1978a).
14. Just because a statement is not known to be
true (false), it does not follow that it is known to
be false (true). An analysis of this fallacy is
given by John Woods and Douglas Walton, "The Fallacy
of *Ad Ignorantiam," Dialectica,* 32, 1978, 87-99.
15. Robert Veatch suggested that I should point
out here that the number of people who have been
falsely pronounced dead by using heart and lung
criteria must exceed by a factor of millions the
number who will ever falsely be pronounced dead using brain-oriented criteria.
16. For further discussion of irreversibility, see
Part Three, fourth section.
17. According to Robert Veatch, however, his notion
of social interaction would include such elementary
interactions as the ability to perceive the presence
of another. He would argue that a situation could
never exist where a person has the capacity to perceive or even be conscious without the capacity to
perceive or be conscious of the presence of another
person. I fail to see why such a situation could
not exist, so perhaps we disagree on this point, or
at any rate do not use "capacity to perceive" or
"be conscious of the presence of another" in the
same way.

Glossary of Medical Terms

Angiography. A diagnostic tool used to determine the status of the blood vessels or lymphatic system.

Anoxia. The absence of oxygen in arterial blood or tissues.

Blood-brain barrier. The cerebral capillary walls do not allow various substances to pass across them. These substances are not exchanged between the blood and the brain. This is an important protective mechanism for maintaining conditions necessary for optimal brain function.

Brain stem. That part of the brain connecting the cerebral hemisphere to the spinal cord.

Cardiorespiratory (cardiopulmonary). Relating to the heart and lungs.

Cephalic (cranial). Relating to the head.

Cerebrum. The largest portion of the brain consisting of the two cerebral hemispheres.

Cerebral cortex. The outer portion of the cerebral hemispheres.

Central nervous system (CNS). The brain and spinal cord.

Electroencephalograph (EEG). A technique by which the electrical activity of the brain is recorded from leads attached to the scalp.

Hydrocephalus. A pathological condition accompanied by an excessive accumulation of fluid in the brain.

This results in a thinning of the brain and separation of the cranial bones.

Intracranial. Within the cranium or skull.

Lesion. A wound or injury.

Liquefaction. The change from a solid to liquid form form.

Neurologist. A physician specializing in disorders of the nervous system.

Neuron. A nerve cell. The basic functional unit of the nervous system.

Respirator (ventilator). A device for administering artificial respiration for a prolonged period of time.

Reye's Syndrome. A sudden loss of consciousness in children accompanied by cerebral edema and marked fatty changes in the liver and kidney.

Subcortex. A term used in this monograph to denote the brain stem plus the cerebellum, including all the subcortical regions of the brain.

Synapses. The connections through which neurons communicate.

Bibliography

Agich, George J. "The Concepts of Death and Embodiment." *Ethics in Science and Medicine* 3 (1976):
95-105.

Arnold, David. "Neomorts." *University of Toronto
Medical Journal* 54 (1977): 35-37.

Beecher, Henry K. "A Definition of Irreversible
Coma. Report of the Ad Hoc Committee of the Har-
vard Medical School to Examine the Definition of
Brain Death." *Journal of the American Medical
Association* 205 (1968): 337-40.

Beecher, Henry K., and Dorr, Isaiah H. "The New
Definition of Death: Some Opposing Views,"*Inter-
nationale Zeitschrift fur Klinische Pharmakologie,
Therapie und Toxicologie* 5 (1971): 120-24.

Black, Peter M. "Definitions of Brain Death," in
Ethical Issues in Death and Dying. Edited by
Tom L. Beauchamp and Seymour Perlin. Englewood
Cliffs: Prentice-Hall, 1978.

_____. "Brain Death." *New England Journal of Medi-
cine.* Part I, 299 (1978a): 338-45; Part II,
299 (1978a): 393-401.

Capron, Alexander M., and Kass, Leon R. "A Statutory
Definition of the Standards for Determining Human
Death." *University of Pennsylvania Law Review*
121, (1972): 87-118.

Capron, Alexander M. "Legal Definition of Death."
*Brain Death: Interrelated Medical and Social Is-
sues, Annals of the New York Academy of Sciences*
315 (1978): 349-59.

Converse, Ronald. "But When Did He Die?: Tucker V.
Lower and the Brain-Death Concept." *San Diego*

Law Review 12 (1975):   424-35.
Currie, Bethia S.   "The Redefinition of Death," in
    Organism, Medicine and Metaphysics.   Edited by
    Stuart F. Spicker.   Dordrecht: Reidel, 1978.
Grenvik, Ake; Powner, David J.; Snyder, James V.;
    Jastremski, Michael S.; Babcock, Ralph A.; and
    Loughhead, Michael G.   "Cessation of Therapy in
    Terminal Illness and Brain Death."   *Critical Care
    Medicine* 6 (1978):   284-91.
Harp, James R.   "Criteria for the Determination of
    Death."   *Anesthesiology* 40 (1974):   391-97.
Hirsh, Harold L.   "Brain Death: Medico-Legal Fact
    or Fiction?"   *Northern Kentucky State Law Forum* 3
    (1975):   16-41.
Ingvar, David H.; Brun, Arne; Johansson, Lars; and
    Samuelsson, Sven M.   "Survival after Severe Cere-
    bral Anoxia with Destruction of the Cerebral Cor-
    tex: The Apallic Syndrome."   *Annals of the New
    York Academy of Sciences* 315 (1978):   184-214.
Jastremski, Michael; Powner, David; Snyder, James;
    Smith, Jan; and Grenvik, Ake.   "Problems in Brain
    Death Determination."   *Forensic Science* 11 (1978):
    201-12.
Jonas, Hans.   "Against the Stream: Comments on the
    Definition and Redefinition of Death," in *Philo-
    sophical Essays*.   Edited by Hans Jonas, Engle-
    wood Cliffs: Prentice-Hall, 1974.
Kass, Leon R.   "Death as an Event."   *Science* 173
    (1971):   698-702.
Korein, Julius.   Preface to *Brain Death: Inter-
    related Medical and Social Issues*.   *Annals of the
    New York Academy of Sciences* 315 (1978):   1-10.
_____   "The Problem of Brain Death: Development
    and History."   *Brain Death: Interrelated Medi-
    cal and Social Issues*.   *Annals of the New York
    Academy of Sciences* 315 (1978a):   19-38.
Law Reform Commission of Canada.   *Criteria for the
    Determination of Death*.   Working Paper 23, Otta-
    wa, 1979.
Manitoba Law Reform Commission.   *Report on a Statu-
    tory Definition of Death*.   Winnipeg, 1974.
Nagel, Thomas.   "Death."   *Noûs* 4 (1970):   73-80.

Roelofs, Richard. "Some Preliminary Remarks on
   Brain Death." *Brain Death: Interrelated Medi-
   cal and Social Issues. Annals of the New York
   Academy of Sciences* 315 (1978): 39-44.
Saunders, Michael G. "Medico-Legal Aspects of Brain
   Deaths." Vol. XII of *Handbook of Electroencepha-
   lography and Clinical Neurophysiology.* Edited by
   R. N. Harner and R. Nacquet. Amsterdam: Elsevier,
   1974.
Schiffer, R. B. "The Concept of Death: Tradition
   and Alternative." *Journal of Medicine and Philos-
   ophy* 3 (1978): 24-37.
Schwager, Robert L. "Life, Death and the Irrevers-
   ibly Comatose," in *Ethical Issues in Death and
   Dying.* Edited by Tom L. Beauchamp and Seymour
   Perlin. Englewood Cliffs: Prentice-Hall, 1978.
Skegg, P.D.G. "Irreversibly Comatose Individuals:
   'Alive' or 'Dead'?" *Cambridge Law Journal* 33
   (1974): 130-44.
_____. "The Case for a Statutory Definition of
   Death." *Journal of Medical Ethics* 2 (1976):
   190-92.
Stuart, Frank P. "Progress in Legal Definition of
   Brain Death and Consent to Remove Cadaver Organs."
   Surgery 81 (1967): 68-73.
Van Evra, James. "On Death as a Limit." *Analysis*
   31 (1971): 170-77.
Van Till, Adrienne—d'Aulnis de Bourouill. "How Dead
   Can You Be?" *Medicine, Science and the Law* 15
   (1975): 133-47.
_____. "Diagnosis of Death in Comatose Patients un-
   der Resuscitation: A Critical Review of the Harvard Report." *American Journal of Law and Medicine* 2, (1976): 1-40.
_____. "Legal Aspects of the Definition and Diag-
   nosis of Death." *Handbook of Clinical Neurology.*
   Edited by P. J. Vinken and G. W. Bruyn. Vol. 24,
   part II. Amsterdam and Oxford: North-Holland,
   1976a.
Veatch, Robert M. "The Whole-Brain Oriented Concept of Death: An Outmoded Philosophical Formu-
   lation." *Journal of Thanatology* 3 (1975): 13-30.

_____. "The Definition of Death: Ethical, Philo-
sophical, and Policy Confusion." *Brain Death: Interrelated Medical and Social Issues. Annals of
the New York Academy of Sciences* 315 (1978): 307-
21.
_____. *Death, Dying, and the Biological Revolution.*
New Haven and London: Yale University Press, 1976.
Veith, Frank J.; Fein, Jack M.; Tendler, Moses D.;
Veatch, Robert M.; Kleiman, Marc A.; and Kalkines,
George. "Brain Death: A Status Report of Medi-
cal and Ethical Considerations." *Journal of the
American Medical Association* 238 (1977): 1651-55;
and "Brain Death II: A Status Report of Legal Con-
siderations." *Journal of the American Medical As-
sociation* 238 (1977): 1744-48.
Walker, A. Earl. "The Death of a Brain." *Johns Hop-
kins Medical Journal* 124 (1974): 190-201.
Walton, Douglas N. *On Defining Death.* Montreal:
McGill-Queen's University Press, 1978.
White, R. J.; Wolin, L. R.; Massoput, L. C.; Taslitz,
N.; and Verdura, J. "Primate Cephalic Transplantation: Neurogenic Separation, Vascular Association." *Transplantation Proceedings* 3 (1971):
602-4.
Woods, John. *Engineered Death.* Ottawa: University
of Ottawa Press, 1978.

Index